Heart Harmony

"Understanding and living with Heart Disease"

Dr. Ashutosh Kumar
MD DM FACC FHRS

STARDOM BOOKS

www.StardomBooks.com

STARDOM BOOKS

112, Bordeaux Ct, Coppell,

TX 75019, USA.

FIRST EDITION NOVEMBER 2023

STARDOM BOOKS, LLC

112, Bordeaux Ct, Coppell,
Tx 75019, USA.

www.stardombooks.com

Stardom books, United States
Stardom Alliance, India

HEART HARMONY

Dr. Ashutosh Kumar

P. 274
cm. 13.5 x 21.5

Category: Health&Fitness/Diseases-Heart

ISBN: 978-1-957456-35-5

DEDICATION

This book is devoted to:

My Mother

Mother India (The cradle of Human civilization)

Mothers across all generations (Past, Present, and Future)

It acknowledges the spirited nature within each individual, resembling the pulsing heartbeat that breathes life and dynamism into the world that envelops us.

CONTENTS

PREFACE

Welcome to the world of heart health!

Whether you have been diagnosed with heart disease or are curious about the journey our hearts take from health to disease, this book is here to guide and empower you. As a cardiologist, my primary goal has always been to help my patients understand their condition and make informed decisions about their treatment. I firmly believe that knowledge is power, and by demystifying the fear associated with heart disease, we can pave the way for a more harmonious life with curable as well as incurable heart disease.

Before we embark on this enlightening journey together, I would like to take a moment to express my gratitude. This book is dedicated in memory of my dear friend, the late C Kripakar, who taught me the essence of empathy during our school days. He encouraged me to write this book while he battled his heart disease, envisioning it as a resource for patients like him and their families who often encounter confusion in their online searches (Googling) about the disease and its treatment options. Unfortunately, I cannot present this book to my dearest friend who inspired its creation.

I am grateful to my parents (Smt Manna Devi & Sri Ganesh Thakur) for their unwavering support and encouragement throughout my career. Without their love and belief in me, I wouldn't be where I am today. I express my appreciation to Dr. Srinivas Narayan (my elder brother), Mr. G Bhaskar Rao, and Mr. Jaganadha Rao & Dr. Sri Lakshmi for their steadfast encouragement and motivation, continuously urging me to strive for more significant achievements. Furthermore, I thank my life partner, Dr G Bhawani, for her invaluable support in completing this book. Her love for me and commitment to her role as a medical profession educator played a crucial part in inspiring me to undertake this writing journey. I thank my lovely daughter Annanya and son Kartikeya, who have always dedicated their time and efforts to supporting and investing in this noble cause. Their unwavering belief in spreading awareness about heart health has been a constant source of inspiration for me.

I am indebted to all my friends from Kendriya Vidyalaya Kanpur, especially Late Kripakar, Aditya Baruah, Sachin Verma, Bhupal Singh, Ranjiv Sharma, Neeraj Shukla, Ajay Nigam and Mascha Sinha, who never failed to encourage me during the challenging process of securing a medical seat after repeated failures in entrance examinations. They stood as consistent pillars of support. They saw the potential in me even before I became a doctor. I owe a debt of gratitude to my college batchmates, especially Sunil Kumar, Neera Kumari, Ashok Prasad, Ajay Bando, Gaurav Kumar, Atul Gupta, Sant Pandey Manojit Lodha as well as all my seniors, Juniors and all my teachers, especially Dr. Kamlesh Tiwari, Dr. Mantosh Panja, Dr. Amal Banerjee, Dr. Avijit Banerjee, Dr. Arupdas Biswas, Dr. Biswakesh Majumdar, Dr Achyut Sarkar, whose constant encouragement and belief in my abilities have been instrumental in shaping my journey as a cardiologist.

I express my sincere gratitude to Dr. John Mandrola, a globally renowned Cardiologist and Chief Cardiology Consultant at Medscape. He has been my go-to mentor in cardiology, providing unbiased insights through his Medscape platform for doctors, which significantly added value in simplifying some complex patient topics while writing this book.

Thanks to a dedicated team of Stardom publications, Mrs. Ranjitha Vijayakumar, Mr. Raam Anand, Mrs. Rekha Krishnaprasad, Mr. Harshvardhan, and Mr. Tejas HK, and for support throughout the writing process—special thanks to Miss Sumana Ghosh for her wonderful insights while crafting the book.Last but not least, I would like to express my deepest gratitude to all the patients who have entrusted me through their resilience, determination, and unwavering spirit that I have learned the true nuances of medical science. Each patient has taught me invaluable lessons, and I am forever grateful for the opportunity to make a difference in their lives.

I aim to provide you with the necessary information about heart disease and its course in this book. I hope it will empower you to take control of your health, make informed decisions, and embrace the opportunities for treatment. Together, we can navigate the path to a healthier heart and a happier life.

Warm Regards,

Dr. Ashutosh Kumar

MD DM FACC FHRS

Hyderabad India.

October 13, 2023.

SECTION-A

INTRODUCTION

"I love listening to the sound of your heart beating, the comforting memory of a cuddling womb."

- Adiela Akoo

Romantics and Cardiologists disagree on most things- mainly because each belongs to a different discipline. But there is one thing that both agree on unanimously: The importance of the heart in a person's life. Whether you are a romantic or not, you are born into this world with one heart and married to it for life. If you want to look at it that way, it's your first arranged marriage. Like your spouse, your heart is the most essential part of your life and the interior center of your body. All the other organs have to dance to the tune of your heart, which is its heartbeat. The Human Heart is the most critical autonomous organ in our body.

Unfortunately, most people are unaware of how the most crucial organ of the human body functions and the growing complexities it can have. But, the recent phenomenon of young adult deaths created widespread fear and anxiety among people. There were also several misconceptions and flawed rumors. It warrants a sensible response from the medical community. As a cardiologist with two decades of experience in both the domain of cardiology- interventional (angiography stenting, valve replacement). As well as electrophysiology (pacemaker, arrhythmia), I am taking this opportunity to address the facts related to heart diseases and dispel rumors. Through this book, I wish to diffuse those fears that have rampantly been propagated to run particular health businesses on false premises. I also want to create better awareness among the general public about identifying heart disease at its outset and reaching out to the doctor for better treatment. For those of you currently suffering from heart ailments, this book will offer you a better understanding of your disease, and you will be confident in facing your heart problems boldly and learn to live in harmony with them.

Heart-"An organ never fails to deliver"

The human heart is a unique masterpiece of God's creation. Unlike other organs, it is fully autonomous. The heart is endowed with an electrical system and can maintain its circulation-something that other organs can't do. They need nutrition and electricity from another organ. It pains me to witness people mock this magnificent piece of God's exquisite creation due to ignorance. The Heart is God's creation and, honestly, a fighter organ behaving much like a determined soldier for the nourishment of whole body organs. How God can leave such an organ is vital for survival, defenseless without tools and means to counter adversities. The human heart is an entirely independent organ in the body. It continuously circulates the blood through each part of your body so that each organ can do its work. As any impairment of heart function has a direct and immediate bearing on all the organs, the heart has been endowed with a compensatory mechanism to adapt to maintain its circulation in the most adverse circumstances of hemodynamics, also called **autoregulation**. Such a critical organ needs coronary autoregulation (the capacity of the coronary circulation to alter vascular resistance to maintain a relatively constant blood flow over a wide range of mean arterial pressure (MAP) from 50-150mmHg) in acute hemodynamic instability. Coronary autoregulation is not the only compensatory mechanism to protect the myocardium from hypoxic injury (ischemia).

It can reinforce **collateral circulation** during progressive coronary stenosis (stenosis means block in coronary circulation). The arteriogenesis (sprouting of new arteries) from a pre-existing coronary network in response to progressive compromise in coronary circulation (coronary stenosis/block). It commences when there is progression of the coronary stenosis severity in the recipient artery, leading to the development of new thin vessels that may or may not be visible during an angiogram. These collateral connections between blocked coronary and nearby artery branches provide circulation to the territory of the blocked coronary artery, preserving heart pumping even in the presence of CTO (chronic total occlusion). CTO is a state of a blocked coronary artery for three or more months. The heart is caged inside the chest behind the sternum bone to protect it from external injury and cushioned from either side by the lungs. These miraculous powers (Autoregulation and Collateral circulation) allow the heart to withstand the brunt of injury (inflammation, ischemic injury). It is the repeated brunt of its adaptability over a prolonged time or a heavy blow to its function in a short period when it fails in its highest performance. This is what we call heart failure. But in the true sense, it is not failure; it is impairment of its efficiency. It is still working without rest and indeed in the adverse maladapted state to provide the best circulation to all the organs so that life can go on. When it stops working, we must declare that "the person" has become the "body." As a cardiologist, I know the heart never fails. It dies after fighting the most brutal assaults of hypertension, diabetes, atherosclerosis ischemia, or inflammation. No organ has so much adaptability to function even in a diseased or injured state than the heart. In the coming chapter, you will learn how the heart handles adversity like hypertension, diabetes, inflammation, ischemia, and toxin exposure.

Engagement to Marriage with disease

Let us accept that diseases are a part of life. We attract diseases through genetics, daily habits, environmental factors, and lifestyle. Every individual, including twins, is different regarding disease risk. Some attract easily, while others are immune to old age. Old age is when our body's organ system faces the degenerative phenomenon of changes destined by nature. There are years of degenerative diseases in our personal lives before our body says goodbye to "the person" and becomes "the body." We should be aware that we all have some or other type of seedlings for diseases inside us, which are dictated by our genetic, environmental factors, and lifestyle. This seedling can prop up in a plant or tree at any time if we are not weeding out this seedling related to lifestyle or environment. Anybody can develop a disease depending upon their genetics and lifestyle. Here, we are discussing incurable, lifelong diseases. We have to accept the disease first and then find ways to get better control of the disease. When it is a lifelong disease like hypertension or diabetes, we are married to it. It is always better to know everything in the patient domain related to disease, at least how to live along with the doctor. We should know the habits we have to teach, and at the same time, we should be bold enough to say goodbye to the routine that can accelerate the disease's progression or complication. We need to know the kinds of available medicines and your alternative options. You should know what would happen if you don't take the medicine and when to escalate and reach for a medical intervention. Taking medication and regular follow-ups is the bare minimum in control of these lifelong incurable diseases. Working on our habits and changing lifestyles in a time-sensitive manner certainly prevent complications as well as the progression of the disease. But some people are very negligent in following these simple rules. As doctors, we also miss some time to give enough time and information to the patients. Driven by a moral responsibility, I strive to record all pertinent information that is accessible to the public, crucial for individuals dealing with heart conditions. This effort will empower them to grasp their ailment and coexist harmoniously with it.

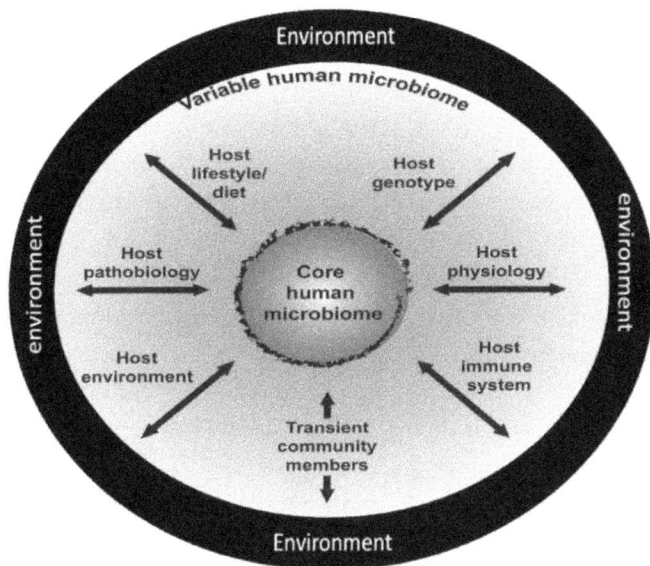

Genesis of Disease

The best description of health and disease is mentioned in Indian text (Ayurveda). We are a microcosm of our environment and exist between our intestines and outside environments.

Whenever there is a loss of harmony between these environments, disease creeps up. The good news is that we have a cure for a handful of diseases. But they are primarily of infectious background. Any disease that is particularly idiopathic or multifactorial risk disease needs to be controlled by medication. These diseases are like pandemic nowadays, which includes hypertension, diabetes, coronary artery diseases, and many more. These diseases are like marriage to somebody enjoying a bachelor's life (healthy life). The unwelcome news of this relationship (married with disease) is that most of the time, there is no option to get out (divorce) of it even if you wanted to, mainly if it is uncurable. It doesn't stop here. If you don't follow the expectations of your new partner (disease) in the form of medicine, diet, exercise, and restrictions, very soon, the partner(illness) will bring home (your body) a toxic sister or other nasty relatives to live with you. It will look like you got married again with other partners(diseases). For example, suppose you have diabetes and are not taking action or control over time. In that case, the chance of getting married to hypertension, coronary artery disease, kidney disease, or eye disease will always be on your card. A harmonious life with one illness prevents many diseases, but denying the first disease invites many diseases and complications. Let me explain how. If you are having atrial fibrillation (a rhythm disorder) and your doctor has diagnosed that, as per the stroke risk scoring, you need an anticoagulant. But denying that they are asymptomatic and don't want any blood thinner or anticoagulant because of bleeding risk then a future event stroke can be taken as an invited problem from your end due to denial of disease like Atrial fibrillation with a high stroke score with premises that you are asymptomatic. We all have the window of opportunity in some diseases called "engagement" with the disease when it has peeped up.

Taking action will prevent it from resulting in marriage or at least postpone the union with the disease from month to year. For example, Studies have proved that if you are obese and at the same time you are developing diabetes (diabetes denovo) or hypertension, an immediate action of 10 % weight loss may reverse your diabetes or hypertension and prevent it for months to years. Hence, managing is discussed in detail in this book, accepting the disease, living in harmony with the disease, and preventing further marriage of the person to another disease wherever possible.

The Evolvement of Complex Diseases

In earlier times, incurable plagues and infections used to spread like wildfire to root out entire communities or villages before people could find some medicine or grow natural immunity. Thankfully, it's not the case anymore. Modern medical advances allow us to control and eradicate many such transmissible deadly infections. Today, most diseases, particularly in the cardiology domain, are non-infectious, and many medications and interventions exist to control them. But we have yet to find a cure for them. We will discuss those in appropriate chapters. At the same time, there are also diseases where medical experts or modern science still couldn't come up with the exact cause (in medical terms, etiology). These can be diagnosed easily on some diagnostic criteria, which can be clinical (patient history and examination) and with lab investigations. But when it comes to cause, we label them as "Idiopathic Diseases. "Diagnosing complex diseases like cancers, cardiac, and autoimmune diseases in the present scenario is not difficult. However, researchers need to find out why it happens to one, not to another, with the same exposure. However, doctors put it aside and move on to treat the patient with whatever generalized medication and treatment is available, hoping it will work. But, "How did the patient acquire that disease?" "What are its causes?" "How can we treat the patient better individually?" These are essential questions that have currently gone out of fashion in the medical profession nowadays. The general public is unaware of this, as doctors usually come up with a general diagnosis, and we treat diseases for a long time without knowing why it happened. Such is the situation even with the most available cutting-edge technology available in medical terminology globally. Let me explain this with an example. If a person develops lung cancer, everybody comes up with the go-to diagnosis of smoking and a few environmental risk factors.

However, about 10% to 20% of patients develop lung cancer without any smoke inhalation. "So, why do those many people who never inhaled smoke in their life develop lung cancer while some chain smokers didn't develop it in their lifetime?" This is only one of those questions that is not being asked or researched correctly, and we must humbly accept that "many unknowns" are still to be discovered. As we cannot make a causal relationship(cause and effect relationship) in most of these incurable diseases, we have solved some of this etiology as multifactorial, polygenic, and the concept of

Framingham Heart Study Begins

1948

1957 — High Blood Pressure and Cholesterol Increase Risk of heart disease

1962 — Smoking Associated With Heart Disease

1967 — Obesity and Physical Activity Associated With Heart disease

1971 — Framingham Offspring Study Begins

1977 — Triglycerides and Lipoproteins Associated With Heart disease

1988 — Isolated Systolic Blood Pressure Directly Associated With Heart disease

1994 — Description of Risk Factors for Atrial Fibrillation

2002 — Framingham Third Generation Study begins

1958   1968   1978   1988   1998   2008...

1961 — The Term Risk Factor Is Introduced

1964 — First Report on Stroke

1970 — High Blood Pressure Increase Risk of Stroke

1974 — Diabetes Associated With Cardiovascular Disease

1978 — Atrial Fibrillation Associated With Stroke

1988 — HDL-C Inversely Associated With Mortality

1996 — Description of Progression From Hypertension to Heart Failure

1998 — Development of New Models to Predict Risk of Coronary Disease

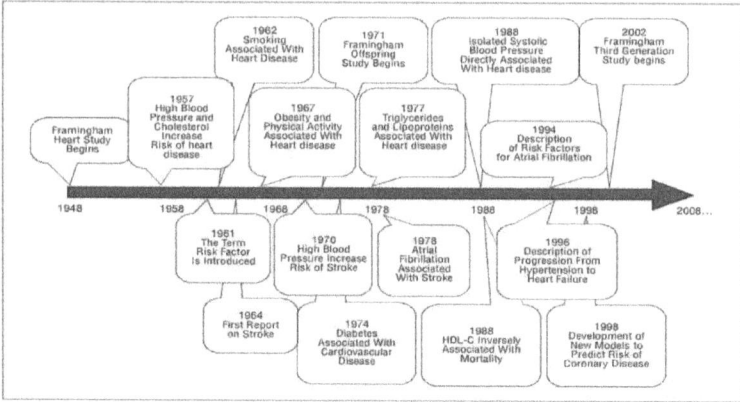

the "risk factors" that can lead to the ailments. Now, we can say smoking is one such risk factor, and so is asbestosis, which means inhaling asbestos. Many "known" risk factors and yet many "unknown" risk factors are yet to be discovered for many cardiac diseases. We will discuss this further in the book. The Framingham study is a landmark study of three generations that started way back in 1948, providing many risk factors for the modern epidemic of coronary artery disease.

However, there is no evidence having a risk factor will lead to disease. By doing trials and studies, we get a glimpse of risk in the population, but answering a specific person is difficult. Over the past two decades, I have seen many such incidences in my practice. Even if you accumulate a risk factor over a long time, the other risk factors will define whether that leads to the disease (some are known and some unknown). And this is how medical science is becoming complex with the evolution of diseases. We need to examine the cumulative risk, which combines all the risk factors with every patient, before developing a wholesome treatment.

Challenging Conditions for Doctors in the Current Medical Environment

In today's world, two things have significantly impacted healthcare delivery for the general public. It is not only the knowledge and skill of a doctor but how well he can walk between the guidelines and medicolegal walls on each side. At the same time, the COPRA (Consumer Protection Act) is meant for the betterment of patients, but patients can't be taken as consumers as it is not business in a true sense. Secondly, for the Indian healthcare system, we do not have our guidelines mindlessly following the US and European guidelines, where everything is insurance or government response. These two changes and the commercialization of the healthcare system have made the healthcare system costly. For example, A patient has visited the hospital's Emergency section with complaints of chest pain. The doctor checks, and it doesn't look like Angina. He performed an ECG, and his baseline ECG was also normal. For this patient, doing Trop T and at least three reports from 1 to 6 hours before releasing them from the hospital becomes mandatory. Yes, Trop T is a good test sensitive as well as specific. However, it cannot be discounted with a good clinical history and risk assessment. Investigations are made to establish diagnosis in addition to our clinical examination. However, the investigation-based approach has taken over the clinical-based approach. "bystander disease" is often treated just on the positivity of some blood marker. For example, if a patient in his 70s who has diabetes, hypertension, chronic kidney disease with COPD due to smoking with cough and nonanginal chest pain but his trop T was mildly positive with echocardiography showing moderate LV dysfunction(LVEF-38%) and underwent angiography showing 80% block in distal LAD and mildly disease in rest two vessel. If he undergoes angioplasty for this lesion, it is not wrong as per the guideline depending on the severity of the block (>70%), but whether that block was cause for the chest pain, which is primarily due to chronic coughing and chest soreness as well as mildly positive TropT is the mark of myocardial disease than myocardial infarction or coronary artery disease. Here, coronary artery disease is a bystander disease; its treatment with cardiac intervention neither adds days to his longevity nor relieves his chest pain. A heart failure treatment and moderation of his COPD medication are enough.

Here comes the role of the medicolegal system. If we are not conducting the TropT test, we are not keeping the possibility of heart attack as a possibility. If the patient dies for any reason in the hospital or at home, the patient party can sue the doctor for negligence. That makes "over-investigation" and more intervention not based on need but on the information of report, which is sometimes "noise, not signal." They are bystander diseases, which most people develop when they have a risk factor. Their intervention never added longevity in the patient other than placebo sense that his coronary block is cleared and now he is prevented from a heart attack. I firmly believe health and education are pillars of the nation. It should be away from a commercial and business angle, and any compromise in quality control of these two premises will heavily affect the nation's growth and health.

Emergence of the Healthcare system to the Healthcare industry

Unfortunately, in one way or another, modern medicines and technologies collude with the Pharma Companies and Medical Corporations. These corporate giants still invest heavily in modern medical technology and want their investment reimbursed with huge profits. So, they keep beating their band about these limited procedures to control the medical environment. The medical practice is confined to interventional medicine's boundaries to favor the investors. This overall effect burdens the patients, who often need the proper treatment. Over time, the bar of diagnosis and intervention has become low. This is just to market products that are "high-cost -low value" products or interventions, sometimes without solid evidence, also called therapeutic fashion.

We cannot create a healthy life by medical interventions. It is a proven fact that you can't change a person's longevity through interventions, particularly in chronic coronary artery disease. However, the same intervention (primary angioplasty) becomes a lifesaving cardiac intervention during acute cardiac emergencies like

Acute Coronary Syndrome (ACS). Besides your genetics, which are not in your control, your lifestyle and diet habits define your longevity. It's the same for cardiac diseases, too. If you can maintain a better lifestyle, you can enjoy a long life without intervention. For that, your lifestyle should include awareness about the disease. For example, if you have hypertension, you must know what to take care of daily. You should know what options are available for you. You should know symptoms needing early medical consultation rather than routine consultation. At the same time, you should be aware of red flag symptoms in hypertension. It is essential to discover how your disease is linked to your parents. On that basis, what will be a risk of developing in your children when they should be screened?

So these are the minor things done regularly and compounded over time, bringing us to chronic heart disease. I am going to discuss this in the book. Also, if you or any of your loved ones are getting a heart procedure done, what will be the prognosis? How can you take care of yourself or them? Things like these, which are not there in the public domain or social media, will also be detailed in this book.

Heart diseases- Fabricated Fears & Misunderstandings

Nowadays, you will find two specific kinds of patients who visit hospitals regarding heart ailments. The first is "overanxious" about getting disease and death, and the second is in "denial mode" for already diagnosed diseases. Either of these modes of thought process is unhealthy. The first kind is those who got anxious after watching the news that some young, healthy celebrity had died from a heart attack during a workout. They searched about it on Google and found confusing information, adding to the anxiety. Some people started labeling physical workout killers, and everybody began doubting exercises. The madness didn't stop there. Businesses and Medicos started encashing their fear. Some Gyms and Clubs also ask their members to produce a health certificate from a doctor or a cardiologist before continuing their exercises. These bizarre norms or guidelines are neither given by any government administration nor medical policies from any of the esteemed bodies of the world (American College of Cardiology/ European Society of Cardiology). But somehow, somewhere, someone kept it in the public domain, and fear started spreading among people. Young people began visiting the hospitals, questioning physical workouts and if there was a chance that they could die doing exercise.

This kind of fabricated fear is not suitable for society. Healthy norms like physical exercise should only be questioned for a strong reason. The reason can be having a history of cardiac disease in the family or genetic disease associated with exercise-related death. But some unrelated celebrity's death shouldn't make everyone jittery about their Heart health. These myths need to be defused so that people can follow healthy norms peacefully without any doubts, and I hope this book helps with that.

The second kind of heart patients reaching hospitals are those with a "denial of the chronic disease ."For example, if a patient is diagnosed with hypertension, many think that all they have is a typical temperament. They are reluctant to accept their blood pressure readings and stop medication alone. They understand I have no symptoms, so why should I have medication? All allopathic medicine has side effects. Why bear these medications? If you somehow convince them to take medication, they stop taking it as soon as their blood pressure normalizes. They are the patient who gets the brunt of this disease, which is silent over some time and finally assaults like a terrorist and damage the vital organ. Its major assault is on the brain, the heart, and the kidneys. It is responsible for 1/3 of deaths globally through stroke or heart attack. Hypertension is again an idiopathic disease and needs more awareness to safeguard its menace. We don't know the exact cause of hypertension in about 95%(Primary Hypertension) of the time. We will again come back to the risk factors based on which we can predict if someone can develop hypertension. Still, even then, we can't be 100% sure as it is a multifactorial disorder, and genetic, lifestyle, and environmental factors play their role, so we have to go case by case.

Another common misunderstanding for patients nowadays is about atherosclerosis and its manifestations. It is a disease where fat gets deposited in the blood vessels, which is an oversimplification of the disease. The disease progression and outcome are complex and multifactorial risk factors. The major arteries of vital organs are essential targets for the disease, and manifestation also depends on the vascular bed involved. It can be anywhere from the affected artery from the brain artery to the toe. The manifestation in the brain(stroke), heart (heart attack), kidney vessel (hypertension & CKD), intestine vessel(bowel gangrene and ischemia), or a lower limb vessel (intermittent claudication or gangrene). Any one of those vessels or any combination of them can be involved in this disease. The limelight is always taken by cardiac and its manifestation because it is most life-endangering while other manifestations are disabling. The heart could be just one of the manifestations of this generalized disease. So, deploying a stent in the coronary artery is a partial treatment. Often, patients and the notion that stenting has cured or wholly controlled the disease need to be corrected. Some patients understand that "Now his disease is cured" by stenting or bypassing. It is the most significant mistake patients make. This misunderstanding has a lot of bearing on the disease progression due to incomplete medical treatment and lifestyle modification, which is equally essential to decelerate the progression of atherosclerosis. The local treatment with a stent or coronary bypass cannot answer this generalized atherosclerosis disease. A generalized illness should be treated in a generalized way. The role of medical management combined with lifestyle modification is the first and foremost treatment, and its role should never be downplayed at any time by the patient or the doctor's team.

Whether it's a heart attack or any other disease, there are a "lot of factors" that have to play their role for a "particular duration" in the timeline to impact the function of the heart, which, in my opinion, is the most evolved organ of human in both functionality and survivalism. The unnecessary fear-mongering around health issues is only helping medical sales rather than public health. The

DANCAVAS study was conducted on the aspect of health packages and evaluation, bringing the prevalent situation to light.

Dancavas Synopsis

EVALUATION- A total of 46,611 participants underwent randomization. The screening included the most advanced investigation, which included non-contrast electrocardiography-gated computed tomography in determining the coronary-artery calcium score and in detecting aneurysms and atrial fibrillation, ankle-brachial blood-pressure measurements to detect peripheral artery disease and hypertension, and a blood sample to see diabetes mellitus and hypercholesterolemia.

RESULT- After more than five years, the invitation to undergo comprehensive cardiovascular screening did not significantly reduce the incidence of death from any cause among men 65 to 74 years of age.

A revelation that has profoundly affected my perspective

Plenty of ambiguous and biased information is propagated about the evaluation of diseases and medical interventions in the present healthcare environment. There needs to be proper conversation or practice of lifestyle modifications in doctor consultations to impact patients' overall health better.

In my personal experience over the last two decades, I found that many things written in medical books are not applicable or partially correct, particularly regarding Indian patients. For example, the literature says that a person who has heart failure with reduced ejection fraction with guideline-directed medication and who had more than two admissions can barely have a chance to survive two years. An ejection fraction in echocardiography reports with heart failure diagnosis differs for all patients. Many factors other than cardiological evaluation play a role in longevity. The last item available in the medical terminology literature is "attitude and mindset" toward the diagnosed disease. A positive mindset and attitude followed by good doctor and patient relationships, medication, proper diet, and exercise deliver the maximum longevity and slightest complication during the journey with these chronic diseases of the heart. My patient experience in my practice was eye-opening and changed how I used to think past those norms and evaluations.

Around 2009, I had just completed my DM (Doctorate of Medicine) and joined a hospital as a cardiologist. One day, an older adult came to me for consultation because he had chest pain. After a preliminary examination, we went for the angiography. He was around 65 and had 20 years of poorly controlled diabetes and a bad lung due to his smoking habit. After we performed the angiography, we found that all three vessels had critical stenosis. One major artery, the LAD (left anterior descending artery), which supplies about 60-70% of the heart, is blocked. We call it CTO (chronic total occlusion) in medical terminology. As per the guideline, he needs coronary bypass surgery as per the anatomy and complexity of coronary stenosis. We thought it was his best option, and I recommended it. After a few days, on the day of surgery, I got an urgent call to visit the operation theatre (OT). It turned out that the patient was not cooperating with the team. I hurried to the theatre. After reaching there, the patient said, "I gave you my consent, thinking that you would operate on me!" Somehow, only I was able to create that trust in him. I explained to the patient that a Cardiologist differs from a Cardiothoracic Surgeon. Cardiologists can only diagnose and treat cardiovascular ailments with medicine or an Interventional procedure like angioplasty and stenting. But operations on the heart, like cardiovascular surgeries, are only performed by Cardiothoracic Surgeons, which is not my domain. The patient was adamant that he wouldn't let anyone else operate on him. He jumped off the operation table and went away. So, finally, we had to cancel his open-heart surgery. A few days later, he returned to consult me at the hospital again, asked for medicines I prescribed for him for the next two weeks, and asked him to see me after two weeks. But he disappeared after that consultation, and I completely forgot about him.

Almost seven years had passed, and the patient returned to me on one fine day. He said to me, "Doctor, do you recognize me?" It took a few minutes for me to recognize him. He was alive and doing well. He had reduced smoking but didn't give up altogether. I was shocked to see such a phenomenon because it was contrary to what I had read and learned through medical books and academics. Our literature says that people in his condition with those many complications can't live long. The difficulties will keep piling up throughout the patient's life, and they will eventually succumb to them. But he did his routine work duties without health complaints or complications. I couldn't believe it! I felt ashamed when he made me remember my words all those years ago: "Doctor, you said that it would be difficult for me to survive without a Bypass Surgery and should be done as early as possible as one is blocked and the other two are critically stenosed." He had proved me wrong. He was still using the same medicines I gave him eight years back and made some modifications to his lifestyle. He was doing most of his field job as a farmer. After that meeting, I followed his condition for five more years as a case study. He was enjoying life with no complications with three hospitalizations (one for chest pain and two for severe cough during corona time) and was seen last time by me in April 2022.

After this experience, I realized that just one ejection fraction in an echocardiogram report won't define a person's life, nor is the chance of a coronary block detected during diagnostics. Doctors should individualize each patient while taking a call on intervention and course of treatment. Several factors are associated with a person's health beyond medicines and interventions. A holistic approach is needed before making conclusions. Each patient is different, allowing us to improve our skills to understand these incurable diseases. Though the generalized norms and guidelines help us to make decisions when the symptoms are not specific to the condition, as in index patients, a case-to-case discussion with treatment options should be taken. From my experience, this can be done with optimal medical management and a better lifestyle and diet. I have seen many similar patients with positive results, but there was one common factor for all these patients. It is their mental attitude towards the diagnosis and its treatment. They were positive throughout the healing process and were not scared by the disease. I have observed that even the medication we prescribe will not work fully if any patient is scared. Eventually, such a patient will need a quick fix of stenting or bypass to relieve the complaints.

This case is not a one-off case. Our professional requirement is such that we need to look at a patient individually on a case-by-case basis. Once in a while, a patient like an index case (the kind of patient described above) appears. That is when we look back and review and try to connect the dots on why some patient develops and showcases fewer symptoms than others who have the same disease and are at a similar stage. When a patient like an index case comes to us, as a cardiologist, we conduct coronary angiography where we can see the blocks and finally recommend either angioplasty or bypass procedure if the blocks are critical. But when we look at the angiography of such a patient, we try to figure things out and start questioning, "Why does the patient have no symptoms or minimal symptoms when all the three vessels are clogged?" The patient's body may have developed a natural bypass, which the coronary angiogram has failed to detect. The resolution of a coronary angiogram is up to 500 microns in diameter. Any coronary or its branch with a width lower than that will be undetected by the coronary angiogram. Hence, this alternative circulation may be why the index patient did not have angina even after working 6-8 hours in the field as a dairy farmer. His condition was severe because he had critical stenosis in 3 coronary arteries, and one was blocked. Such patients may fare better even on medication without any surgery. Even the guideline for medical management recommends that for any chronic coronary artery disease, any intervention should be planned if they remain symptomatic, even on optimal medical control and lifestyle modification.

Book vs. Real Practice

Patients as teachers and books as guides were told to us during college. I have learned a lot and am still learning from each case. In medical science, one plus one is not always two. It can be three, four, five, or even eleven. This means that every patient and case of a disease is unique, and we may always overlook other factors. We must be diligent with each patient and find individualized treatment accordingly. There is no doubt that medical science is a boon for acute medical emergencies where we can fix things immediately and save the patient's life. We can open blocked coronary within minutes, salvage the patient from dying from a heart attack, and revive the heart pumping function. When a patient enters the Cath lab, we can pass a wire and deploy a stent. We have similar intervention procedures for all emergencies. However, when it comes to lifelong diseases, we should educate patients on how to manage them and give them a chance at conservative management without invasive procedures unless it is life-endangering or makes a remarkable change in their long-term prognosis. We should diffuse the fear arising from chronic disease and help them with medication, lifestyle modification, and intervention without bias to any of the mentioned. Unfortunately, this is not happening in the present time of practice in medical science due to both patient and doctor factors.

Therefore, I want to provide this book's most detailed disease-specific information. I want to educate readers on what is good for them and what is bad, how to live happily while managing a disease, how to live with medication and lifestyle changes, and what the dos and don'ts are. The motto of this book is to help readers live in harmony with heart disease, which is diagnosed and found to be incurable, and at the same time, know what options are available for their heart disease.

The practice and experience of doctors should make a difference in society. As a duty to society, I share these pearls about cardiac disease and its treatment before people reach the hospital. There should not be any fallacious fear factors in the public domain that drive people to the hospital unnecessarily. Unfortunately, the opposite is rampant in society nowadays due to the heavy commercialization of the medical field and the business models of hospitals. This book represents a modest endeavor to transcend these commercial obstacles and fulfill the request of a very dear friend, the Late C. Kripakar, who requested me to present my knowledge of cardiology so that if ever someone develops the disease, they will have a picture of their subsequent journey with the disease. This book will help empower the reader with helpful information and genuine insights into heart health and how to live harmoniously with cardiac ailment. The knowledge within is drawn from my two decades of experience in cardiology.

1

THE HEART: YOUR INCREDIBLE BIOLOGICAL MOTOR

"The heart has its reasons of which reason knows nothing."

- Blaise Pascal

The heart is a symbol of life. It beats with its rhythmic pulse, a core indicator of life, and its absence signifies death. It's astonishing to know that the beginning of a new life and the initiation of the heartbeat occur on the 22nd day after fertilization within the mother's womb. This marks the inception of an extraordinary biological motor that will tirelessly serve new human beings throughout their lifetime. Initially, the heart forms as a small tubular embryonic structure, rapidly growing into a complex, four-chambered organ.

The Heart's Function: The heart is a robust and persistent motor that propels the incredible vehicle of the human body. Blood carries the essential ingredients needed for metabolism and nourishment. It works as fuel and a medium for transporting different ingredients between the organs. The heart's primary function is to pump blood to all organs. The heart and its connection with other organs through the artery originating from the main trunk (aorta), a vessel from the heart guarded by the aortic valve to provide forward flow when the heart ejects blood in the aorta. These arteries penetrate the vessel and ramify into the arteriole and the capillary bed. This capillary bed, which is one cell width, is the site of the exchange of blood ingredients. The exchange will happen according to gradients and needs. Then, these capillaries convert into existing vessels called venules. Finally, veins exit the organ after nourishing it and returning its excreted material to the mainstream trunk line. These trunk lines that flow towards the heart and carry the blood after nourishing the organ are called vena cava. They finally drain in the heart's upper chamber, the right atrium. The heart and vessels are called the cardiovascular system. The heart has a unique function of circulating blood throughout the entire body and simultaneously to itself. It pumps the blood to all organs, we call it systole (the contraction phase), and fulfills its needed blood supply during diastole(relaxation phase). Unlike other organs, the heart is an autonomous entity, independent and automatic in functioning. Unlike other muscles, it is not dependent on the brain for its contraction. That's why brain

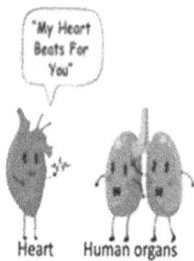

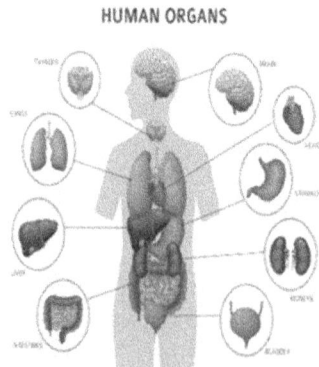

HUMAN ORGANS

Heart   Human organs

death cannot be equated to heart death. It is an independent organ that maintains the human body's survivability by providing circulation to all organs and sustaining the life of all other organs by providing them with oxygen and nutrients through blood circulation. It operates continuously without rest until our final breath.

The Heart's Electrical System: Its remarkable electrical system is Central to the heart's operation. At the junction of the right upper chamber (right atrium) and the superior vena cava, a structure known as the sinoatrial node (SA node) serves as the heart's electrical generator. That is the reason the normal rhythm is called *sinus rhythm*. It pulsates and generates electrical impulses that travel through specialized channels within the heart muscle, causing its contraction. The SA node provides the autonomy of heart electrical activity by a unique channel in the cell membrane known as *the funny channel*. The generated current is called *If current*, initiating and perpetuating the heart's continuous beating. This current provided by *the funny channel* in the SA node gives the unique automaticity and provides the heart with its source of electricity.

The Electrical Pathway: From the SA node, the electrical impulses flow directly to the left upper chamber through an electrical bundle called Bachmann's bundle. Simultaneously, three internodal tracts within the right upper chamber facilitate the transmission of impulses to the atrioventricular node (AV node). This AV node is a vital structure located at the junction of the heart's four chambers and at the apex of *Koch's triangle* in the right atrium. The AV node acts as a crucial *Transmitter of the heart*, supplying the current generated by the SA node (*electrical generator of the heart*) to the lower chambers(ventricle). An electric bundle known as the His bundle originates from the AV node and then descends along the wall separating the two lower chambers(*ventricle*) called interventricular septum into right and left branches called right bundle branch (RBB) and left bundle branch (LBB). They further ramify into Purkinje fibers to finely innervate cardiac muscle(ventricle). This intricate pathway ensures the coordinated contraction and relaxation of the heart chambers, resulting in the familiar rhythm of the heartbeat.

Anatomy and Functioning of the Heart: The heart, often described as the size of a closed fist and weighing approximately 280 to 350 grams, consists of four chambers, each equipped with a valve. The two upper chambers, called atria, receive blood, while the lower chambers, known as ventricles, pump blood out of the heart. The right atrium collects impure or venous blood from all organs via two primary veins: the superior vena cava (from the upper body) and the inferior vena cava (from the lower body). This blood flows through the tricuspid valve into the right ventricle. Upon contraction, the right ventricle ejects the blood through the pulmonary valve into the pulmonary arteries, transporting it to the lungs for purification. The oxygenated and purified blood returns to the left atrium through the four pulmonary veins. From the left atrium, the blood enters the left ventricle through the mitral valve. During ventricular systole, the left ventricle propels the oxygenated blood through the aortic valve into

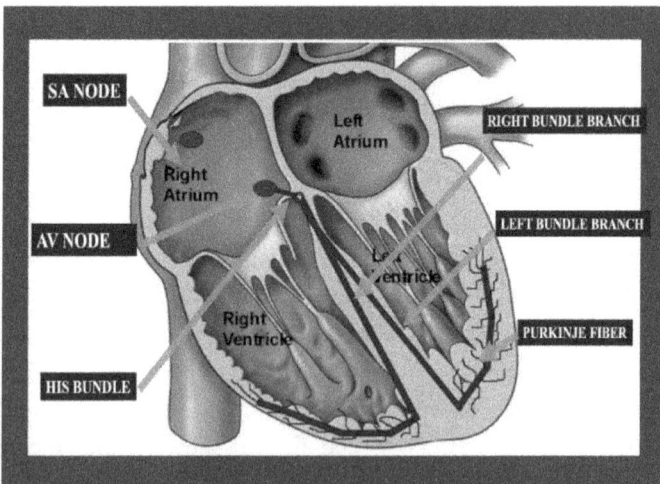

the aorta, distributing it to the entire body. The heart's diastole phase allows the ventricles to relax and refill with blood from the atria, preparing for the next contraction.

The Heart's Unique Circulation: Think of your heart as a pump that works non-stop to send blood to all body parts. But even the heart needs its supply of blood to stay healthy and function properly. That's where the coronary arteries come in. These unique blood vessels start from the main blood vessel called the aorta and give the heart the oxygen and nutrients it needs to stay strong. This happens during diastole.

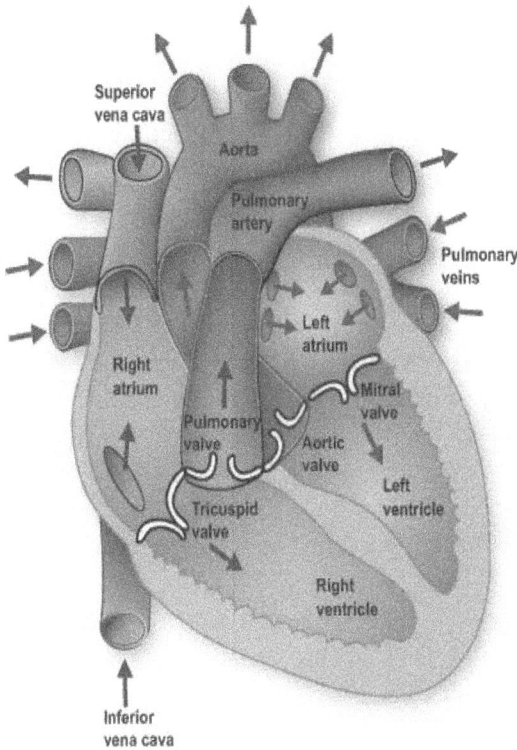

Circulatory System of the Heart

Now, just like how the heart has its blood supply, it also has a way to get rid of used-up blood. This is where the coronary veins come in. The greater, middle, and smaller cardiac veins collect the blood that the heart doesn't need anymore and bring it back to the heart's right side. These veins combine to make a bigger vein called the coronary sinus, which acts like a drain for all the used-up blood from the heart. This coronary sinus is like a bridge between the heart's upper (left atrium) and lower left chambers (left ventricle). It drains the blood into the right atrium.

This coronary sinus becomes essential when trying to help people with heart problems. We use it in cardiac resynchronization therapy of the heart to make it work better during cases of heart failure. The coronary sinus helps the heart's left side work together with the right side, essential for people with heart failure.

As an incredible biological motor, the heart powers the human body with its continuous, rhythmic beating. Its autonomous nature, electrical system, and complex anatomy enable it to sustain life by providing oxygen and nutrients to all organs. Understanding the intricacies of the heart's functioning and maintaining its health is essential for a fulfilling and active life. In the subsequent chapters, we will delve deeper into various aspects of heart health, dispel myths, and provide practical guidance on managing heart ailments and fostering a harmonious relationship with your heart.

The Circulatory System of the Human Body: The heart cannot be discussed without considering the circulatory system, also known as the cardiovascular system. It consists of the heart, the network of blood vessels, and the blood itself. Blood is often referred to as a liquid tissue and serves as the fuel that sustains every cell in our body. With an estimated 37 trillion cells forming various organs and body parts, each cell requires oxygen and nutrients to perform its specific functions. The circulatory system fulfills this need by delivering oxygen-rich blood, carrying hemoglobin and nutrients such as carbohydrates, proteins, fats, vitamins, minerals, different metabolites, and water to every cell with each heartbeat.

The circulatory system comprises two distinct types of blood vessels: (Arteries and Veins). Arteries carry oxygenated blood away from the heart to the organs and cells of the body, while veins transport deoxygenated blood back to the heart. The journey begins with the heart's left ventricle ejecting purified blood into the aorta, the primary artery. From the aorta, branches called the ascending and descending aorta supply oxygenated blood to different regions. At the aortic arch, three arteries branch out to deliver purified blood to the upper parts of the head, including the brain. The descending aorta further branches into numerous arteries, ensuring that purified blood reaches the lower parts of the body. The blood, enriched with oxygen, travels from the heart through the aorta, arteries, and arterioles and eventually reaches micro-sized capillaries present in all organs. In these capillaries, the exchange of oxygen and nutrients occurs, nourishing the organs. Deoxygenated blood then returns from the organs through venules into veins and ultimately to the superior and inferior vena cava, which transport it back to the heart's right atrium. The blood circulation follows a branching order of vessels throughout the body. This circulation, which starts from the aorta and ends in the vena cava, is called *systemic circulation*. It is a pressure system, and what we measure our blood pressure is the pressure of systemic circulation.

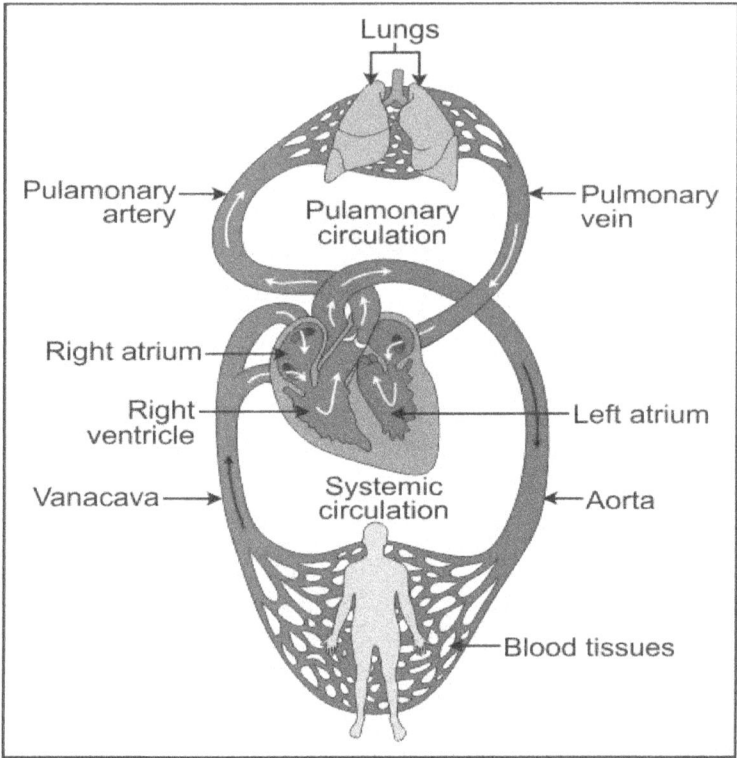

However, pulmonary circulation includes a unique set of blood vessels called pulmonary arteries and pulmonary veins. This is unlike other arteries and veins; their role differs. The pulmonary artery carries deoxygenated blood from the heart's right ventricle to the lungs for purification. In contrast, pulmonary veins are the only vein that transport oxygenated blood from the lungs to the heart's left atrium. This distinction arises because arteries carry blood away from the heart, and veins bring blood back to the heart. Furthermore, the lungs have their oxygen supply through bronchial arteries, which branch separately from the descending aorta to support their functioning.

The circulation between the pulmonary artery and the pulmonary vein is called the pulmonary circulation. They are low-pressure and high-capacitance systems and are not accessible directly for their pressure measurement. An echocardiogram can indirectly measure pressure while invasively measuring pressure by deploying the catheter in the heart. This pulmonary circulation has given our heart an advantage for escalating the oxygen enrichment and removal of carbon dioxide without straining it as it is a low-pressure system. In athletes, the oxygen requirement and carbon dioxide removal from blood require about 20 times over the resting state, which is done by increasing the cardiac output by 4-8 times while taking advantage of this low-pressure high capacitance system. These two systems- pulmonary and systemic circulation- are connected in a series. This association of systemic and pulmonary systems is affected in some congenital heart diseases where it can become parallel, and immediate surgery or intervention is required during neonatal life to save the baby.

Regarding the oxygen levels in the blood, it's important to note that blood always contains some oxygen level, contrary to common belief. Oxygen is carried by hemoglobin within the blood. When we inhale air, the lungs extract oxygen from the inhaled air and saturate hemoglobin with it while simultaneously expelling carbon dioxide. As a result, the oxygenated blood with high oxyhemoglobin levels is transported from the lungs to the heart through pulmonary veins. It then flows through arteries to supply oxygen to organs throughout the body. Each organ draws the required oxygen, depleting the hemoglobin's oxygen level but maintaining a minimal threshold to sustain its status as oxyhemoglobin. When this threshold is unmet, the blood becomes deoxygenated and returns to the lungs through the heart to undergo further oxygenation. Did you know which organ draws the maximum oxygen? It is your brain. It is totally dependent on glucose for its metabolism, and without oxygen, it cannot break glucose to its energy unit called ATP (adenosine Tri Phosphate), the currency of energy. Hence, any derangement of circulation to the brain, even for 10 – 30 sec, is enough to make a person unconscious, mainly if it affects RAS (Reticular Activating System), which lies in the brain stem. Its continuous activation is needed to remain in the conscious state.

Beyond its role in oxygen through red blood cells (Erythrocytes) and nutrient delivery, blood also carries waste products from organs to be processed by the kidneys and liver. Moreover, it protects the body against infections through white blood cells(leucocytes) and blood coagulation with platelets(thrombocytes). The circulatory system functions continuously, fueling cellular energy production and eliminating waste products, thus enabling the body to operate harmoniously.

Evolution of Heart Diseases

Understanding the evolution of heart diseases is crucial in comprehending heart health. Heart diseases can be broadly classified into two main categories: *congenital* heart diseases and *acquired* heart diseases.

Congenital heart diseases are present from birth and are characterized by abnormalities in the structure or functioning of the heart. During the early stages of intrauterine development, the earliest fetal heart-beating activity can be noticed around the 22nd day of intrauterine life, corresponding to the 36th day of gestation. It is not the same mature beat that pushes the blood into great vessels. Abnormality in this process or subsequent growth stages can lead to congenital heart diseases. Examples include abnormalities in the number of heart chambers, holes in the chambers (atrial septal defect, ventricular septal defect, patent ductus arteriosus), or narrowed valve defects (aortic stenosis, pulmonary stenosis). These abnormalities can result from genetic factors, maternal drug use, or disruptions during heart development. Although present at birth, symptoms of congenital heart disease can present themselves from the neonatal phase (first 28 days of life) to childhood, and sometimes it may in adult or old age too manifest later in life. The age of presentation in congenital heart disease depends on many factors. For example, severe valve issues and connections of abnormal circulation usually present in the early part of life, while abnormal valves like the bicuspid aortic valve and ASD, which do not affect the function of the heart adversely, present later in life or as a chance finding during cardiac evaluation for other cause. The diagnosis of PSVT, WPW syndrome (abnormal electrical connection), Long QT syndrome, and Brugada syndrome are also present since birth but manifest at different phases of life. These electrical abnormalities are not usually considered congenital heart disease as they are present in structurally normal hearts. They are congenital electrical diseases.

Acquired heart diseases, however, are not present at birth but develop over time. They can result from infections, lifestyle, and multifactorial factors, including genetic predispositions. Rheumatic heart disease is commonly acquired in childhood or early adulthood. It affects the heart valves, presenting with symptoms of joint complaints and fever, but affects valves at its outset. The disease may take years to a decade to manifest with symptoms of heart disease, and the mitral valve is most commonly affected. Acquired heart diseases also include coronary artery disease (CAD), primarily an idiopathic inflammatory vascular disease affecting most major arterial systems from brain to toe. This vascular inflammation is a multifactorial polygenic disorder, so-called atherosclerosis. Atherosclerosis refers to the deposition of fat inside the major arteries, and the process starts during the 2nd decade of life. It is a smoldering disease that progresses, obstructing or narrowing blood flow in the artery it affects. When this occurs in the coronary arteries supplying the heart, it leads to CAD. Risk factors for atherosclerosis include hypertension, diabetes, dyslipidemia, smoking, sedentary habits, and genetic factors. CAD can present with symptoms such as chest pain (angina), stroke, or transient ischemic attack (TIA) if it affects brain circulation, secondary hypertension if it affects renal circulation, or peripheral artery disease (PAD) with lower limb pain. They are responsible for many erectile dysfunction(ED) cases when it affects the penile artery. The manifestation of atherosclerosis varies depending on the affected blood vessels.

Degenerative heart diseases are the category of acquired heart diseases, which are considered to be age-related changes in the heart. They develop over time due to factors such as stress on valves, calcium deposits, and sclerosis (deposition of fibrous tissues) around vital structures of the heart, affecting their function. The aortic valve is a common brunt of these degenerative changes as it is placed between the aortic valve and left ventricle, a very high-pressure gradient during diastole. The narrowing of the aortic valve, called aortic stenosis, is one of the common degenerative heart diseases. The degenerative diseases predominantly affect the left side valves of the heart, including the aortic and mitral valves, due to their exposure to higher pressure. These degenerative heart diseases can be influenced by age alone or a combination of age and other risk factors.

Understanding the evolution and classification of heart diseases is crucial for effectively managing heart health and preventing complications. In the subsequent chapters, we will delve deeper into these diseases and their risk factors, prevention, and management strategies.

Diseases Related to Heart Muscles & Electrical System: Apart from diseases affecting the heart valves and blood vessels, two other categories of heart diseases commonly affect the heart's muscles and electrical system: arrhythmias and cardiomyopathy.

Arrhythmias refer to diseases where the heart's electrical system is affected, resulting in a change in the rhythm. On the other hand, cardiomyopathy specifically pertains to diseases involving the weakening, dysfunction, or inefficiency of the heart muscles.

Cardiomyopathy can be classified into two common variants. Dilated cardiomyopathy is characterized by an enlargement or dilation of the heart chambers, leading to a decrease in chamber thickness and, ultimately, heart failure. The exact causes of cardiomyopathy are often unknown (idiopathic), but studies suggest that a combination of past viral illnesses and autoimmune phenomena may weaken the heart muscles over time. Dilated cardiomyopathy can be the destination of all heart diseases, from acquired to congenital and from valvular to cardiovascular diseases. They are called secondary cardiomyopathy, which can have dilated chambers and impaired pumping function (reduced ejection fraction) but not primarily due to heart muscle weakness.

Hypertrophic cardiomyopathy, the second variant of cardiomyopathy, involves an increase in the thickness of the heart muscles without hypertension or valve dysfunction. As the muscle mass increases, the size of the heart chamber decreases. This condition occurs in gene abnormality responsible for cardiac muscle contraction.

They are responsible for a fair number of sudden cardiac deaths, particularly in athletes. Patients with hypertrophic cardiomyopathy may experience symptoms such as dyspnea (breathlessness) and palpitations sometimes but may be relatively asymptomatic in many. This thickening of the heart muscle is a significant cause of sudden death in young individuals and often runs in the family. However, it is essential to note that not all athletes should be concerned, as hypertrophic cardiomyopathy has a different prognosis depending on the morphology of the heart and associated genes. Hence, it needs to be individualized during evaluation and treatment. Genetic evaluation of index patients, along with family evaluation, is essential for identifying individuals at risk and implementing appropriate precautions.

Moving on to diseases related to the heart's electrical system, they can be either congenital or acquired. Congenital electrical problems arise from abnormal connections*(pathways)* between the upper and lower chambers of the heart. These pathways between the upper and lower chambers provide alternative parallel connections in the heart. This normal conduction of electricity and abnormal connection(pathway) provides a vicious circuit that can lead to the heart beating very fast. These vicious electrical circuits get activated unpredictably, leading to a very fast heartbeat (150-240/min) at rest and without any reason. This condition is called paroxysmal supraventricular tachycardia (PSVT). Although generally not life-threatening, they can contribute to sudden unbearable palpitation with a feeling of doom when combined with other heart disorders. The elderly patient can have giddiness and fall due to this PSVT, unlike palpation in young patients. Another type of congenital electrical problem involves conduction abnormalities. In this case, the conduction of electricity (impulse) from the upper chamber to the lower chamber is disrupted at the level of *the AV node (transmitter of the heart)* and is called congenital heart blocks. Here, some beats generated at *the SA node (generator of the heart)* fail to reach the lower chambers. This can lead to a very slow heart rate and inadequate blood pumping by the heart, leading to the symptoms of giddiness, syncope, and effort intolerance. These conditions are known as conduction abnormalities.

Acquired electrical problems can develop due to various risk factors and degenerative changes. Abnormal substrates or scars may form within the heart due to the repair of heart injury or inflammation. These abnormal substrates work like volcanos for arrhythmia over time. They can give rise to ectopic beats (Ventricular premature beats), which can be asymptomatic to symptomatic. They can also lead to life-threatening arrhythmia called *ventricular tachycardias (VT) or ventricular fibrillation (VF)*, which compromises heart function. If not attended to urgently, it can kill the person in a fraction of a minute. They are highly disruptive to cardiac pump function, which supplies blood to the body and itself. Rapid and irregular heartbeats characterize ventricular tachycardias, while ventricular fibrillation involves chaotic and ineffective contractions. These life-threatening rhythm disorders can cause sudden cardiac arrest and even death. Symptoms may include dizziness, syncope (fainting attacks), or collapse, requiring immediate medical attention.

Arrhythmias or rhythm disorders can present with a range of symptoms, which are not limited to typical chest pain. In cases where patients experience syncope and collapse, it is likely indicative of an electrical problem in the heart. Prompt diagnosis and appropriate management are crucial for addressing these conditions and preventing potentially life-threatening complications.

2

HOW TO IDENTIFY CARDIOVASCULAR DISEASE (SYMPTOMS & RISK FACTORS)?

"When the heart speaks, the mind finds it indecent to object."

-Milan Kundera

Daily, we experience many symptoms, from simple headaches to leg pain. Some symptoms may be mild and inconsequential, while others can be more serious and significant. As doctors, we need to understand and differentiate between these symptoms. It can sometimes be a complex and confusing task. This becomes especially crucial in heart health, as the heart is one of the body's vital organs.

The cardiovascular system is comprised of the heart and all the artery systems functioning in flowing the blood to the organ and the venous system, which reverses the blood from the organ. These organs function in harmony, at least in the distribution of blood. There is no fight for reserving it for them, and the heart is unique in that it takes care to provide circulation even in an injured state like myocardial infarction and inflammation. It always keeps doing its job. All organs are interconnected by the vascular system (artery, vein, and capillary). Any dysfunction that affects the heart indirectly and, at the same time, heart function can compromise the role of these organs. It needs special mention for four vital and closely related organs: The lung (pulmonary system), gut (digestive system), brain (nervous system), and kidney(nephrology). It is not unusual to get symptoms of breathlessness due to the pooling of blood in the lungs and making it heavy when we take a breath. We call it dyspnoea on exertion (DOE). The same pooling of blood happens in the gut, and the intestine gets congested, leading to abdominal fullness, early satiety, heartburn (dyspepsia), and loss of appetite. This finding we called backward failure symptom happens due to congestion of the organs due to the pooling of blood in the organ. It leads to symptoms from that organ, which may appear that the organ is diseased, but it is a symptom of the heart per se. Some findings will happen in the condition of forward failure of heart function. For example, what do you think will happen to a vital organ like the kidney if it doesn't receive blood for purification? It will go into hypotension or shock-like state in acute illness. This leads to decreased urination, and urine function can shut down. Medically, we call them Oliguria and Anuria, respectively. Here, the symptom of the heart is mimicking a kidney problem.

Similarly, a transient decrease of blood to the brain, particularly the midbrain region called the Reticular activating system(RAS), responsible for maintaining the person's consciousness, can lead to unconsciousness. As the patient loses consciousness, it may seem like a brain issue. But this is deceptive because the root of the problem lies in the heart. Many fainting episodes (syncope) remain under-evaluated because they remain in consultation with the neurology domain. The heart is the central organ in circulation, and its symptoms are not related directly but indirectly to the backward pressure effect on the lungs and gut and the forward impact on the brain and kidney.

Let's explore the most common symptoms related to heart

health and gain a deeper understanding of them to distinguish them from harmless sensations.

1. Angina/Cardiac Pain:

Chest pain is the most widely recognized and discussed heart-related symptom. It is also often the primary indicator of a heart attack. People can also experience chest pain triggered by gastric issues or physical strain. Cardiac pain arising from the heart feels distinctively different. But if we pay close attention to the kind of pain that a person is experiencing, we will be able to distinguish them. While other causes, such as gastric issues or physical strain, can trigger chest pain, cardiac pain arising from the heart feels distinctively different if we pay attention to it.

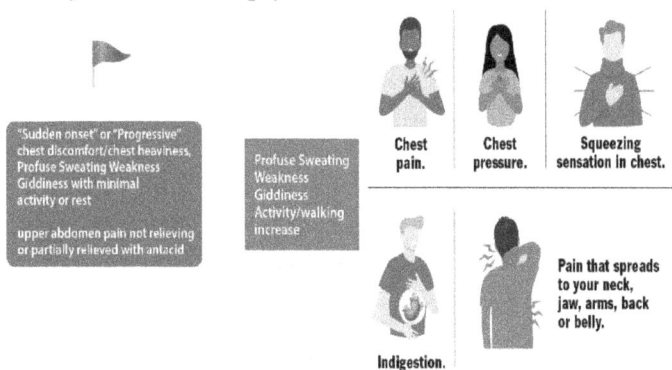

"Sudden onset" or "Progressive" chest discomfort/chest heaviness, Profuse Sweating Weakness Giddiness with minimal activity or rest

upper abdomen pain not relieving or partially relieving with antacid

Profuse Sweating Weakness Giddiness Activity/walking increase

Chest pain.

Chest pressure.

Squeezing sensation in chest.

Indigestion.

Pain that spreads to your neck, jaw, arms, back or belly.

Cardiac **Chest Pain and Angina (Red Flag Sign)** d supply and demand mismatch to the heart. The pain typically starts in the front of the chest, more like heaviness or a feeling of weight on the chest, and this sensation can radiate up to the jawline and down up to the umbilicus. It commonly also radiates to the left arm and sometimes even the back of the chest. This chest sensation(Angina) is different as it cannot be pinpointed on the chest wall like a localized spot but is felt diffusely over the chest. Interestingly, the pain worsens during physical activity like walking and eases or remains stable when the individual rests.

It may happen resting with profuse sweating and extreme weakness, which can be a sign of heart attack (*acute coronary syndrome*). Moreover, the person may experience a sense of impending doom in an acute state as the heart communicates with the brain through numerous nerves, sending warning signals of serious issues.

In some cases, individuals who recognize the symptoms of Angina may self-administer nitrate medication under their tongue to alleviate the pain. If Angina occurs during a resting state without any physical activity, it can be an early warning sign of an impending heart attack, and immediate medical attention is crucial.

Elder (more than 65), elderly, and diabetic patients may not experience typical anginal chest pain. They can have angina equivalents in the form of shortness of breath, nausea, or fatigue that is out of proportion to the activity level. They may encounter abdominal heaviness, bloating sensations, or discomfort just after meals (within 2 hours), and it intensifies if they try to walk just after meals. Often, these individuals might use antacids for gastric relief without realizing their symptoms could be linked to their heart health. The heart needs to pump a significant amount of blood into the intestine after meals to help the intestine digest food. This postprandial increase in cardiac output leads to stress on cardiac circulation if there is a significant block in the coronary circulation. This can present more as abdominal discomfort and chest heaviness, which might be mistaken for a gastrointestinal issue. Heavier meals are higher and longer the duration of this complaints. Recognizing such symptoms as a coordinated manifestation of a heart circulatory issue is vital.

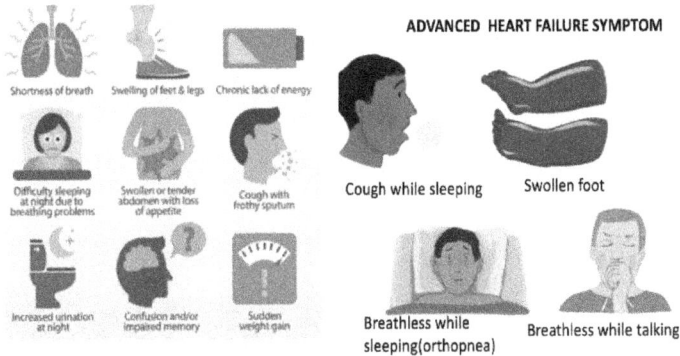

Shortness of breath | Swelling of feet & legs | Chronic lack of energy

Difficulty sleeping at night due to breathing problems | Swollen or tender abdomen with loss of appetite | Cough with frothy sputum

Increased urination at night | Confusion and/or impaired memory | Sudden weight gain

ADVANCED HEART FAILURE SYMPTOM

Cough while sleeping | Swollen foot

Breathless while sleeping(orthopnea) | Breathless while talking

> **Heart Failure**
> **Symptoms**

2. Breathlessness(*dyspnea*):

Shortness of breath (SOB) when happening on exertion, called dyspnea on exertion (DOE), is another critical symptom related to heart disease and can be considered an angina equivalent. In this case, individuals experience labored breathing, as if they are panting for air, even during routine activities that were once effortless. This type of breathlessness can occur when the heart's pumping ability diminishes, or a valve becomes dysfunctional. Additionally, it might be linked to coronary artery disease, where blockages in the coronary arteries restrict blood flow to the heart and compromise cardiac pumping function.

It is essential to differentiate between breathlessness from the heart and the lungs. Individuals who smoke or experience repeated cough and cold symptoms may have respiratory-related breathlessness. In contrast, other cardiac symptoms like chest pain or swelling of the feet often accompany heart-related breathlessness. For those already diagnosed with heart conditions, such breathlessness may indicate the need for further evaluation and prompt medical attention. Breathlessness can happen if the patient is deficient in hemoglobin level(anemia).

An echocardiogram (Echo) is one of the critical investigations performed by expert doctors to diagnose heart-related issues. This test allows visualization of heart chambers, valve function, pumping capacity, and coronary-related issues. Together with other parameters like ECG, the Echo provides invaluable information for accurate diagnosis or ruling out a heart-related complaint.

3. Fatigability:

Fatigability, or the tendency to experience fatigue easily, is characterized by weakness or exhaustion during simple activities that one performs typically effortlessly. This can be an early symptom of a heart disease, particularly issues with heart valves or heart muscles. If a person feels excessively fatigued while attempting simple tasks, it could be indicative of an underlying heart condition. Early diagnosis, particularly for those with a genetic predisposition to heart problems, can be immensely beneficial in managing and treating the condition effectively.

4. Palpitation:

Ordinarily, we remain blissfully unaware of the sound of our heartbeat. But when you hear your heartbeat loud and clear, you need to be attentive to it. The third heart-related symptom that warrants our attention is palpitations. When someone with an underlying heart condition becomes anxious or nervous, their heart may beat rapidly, slowly, or irregularly. The individual begins to feel the pounding sensation of their heartbeat. Often, after a long walk up the stairs or an intense run, you might feel the pounding beat of your heart in your chest—this sensation is known as palpitation. If palpitations occur without any provocation, meaning without extreme physical activity or stress, they should be treated as abnormal and could indicate an underlying heart disease.

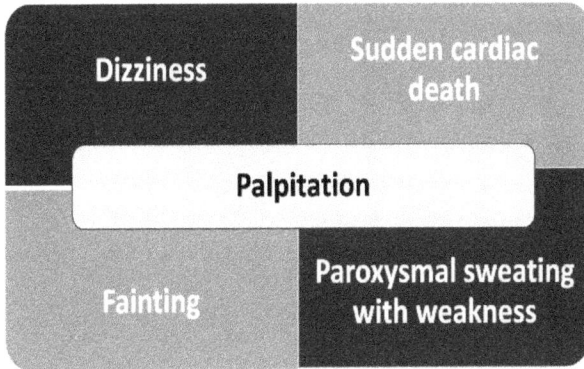

Dizziness	Sudden cardiac death
Palpitation	
Fainting	Paroxysmal sweating with weakness

Symptoms of Arrhythmia (Electrical Problem) or Heartbeat Problems

These palpitations can occur even when the person is sitting still, suddenly experiencing a pounding sensation. Such palpitations are pathological, suggesting an underlying health condition that needs evaluation and diagnosis. There are many reasons why palpitations occur. It can be attributed to heart-related issues like electrical problems, valvular abnormalities, or muscular concerns. Advanced medical tests, including an ECG, can help pinpoint the cause and determine the most appropriate action. It is essential to differentiate cardiac-related palpitations from other reasons to ensure timely and accurate diagnosis.

In some cases, palpitations may also be associated with dizziness, followed by a collapse or syncope, and a family history of sudden deaths. This type of situation warrants heightened concern and urgency as it may be an early warning sign of a potential sudden cardiac arrest. Despite recovering from such episodes, individuals with a family history of sudden cardiac events should undergo a thorough heart-related evaluation to assess potential risks and identify appropriate preventive measures.

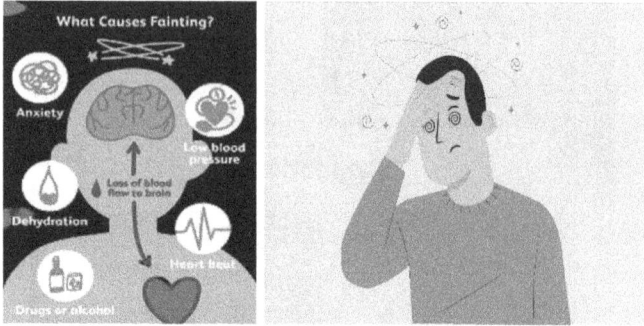

Syncope - A Symptom of Circulation Manifesting from Brain

5. Syncope (fainting):

Syncope refers to the loss of consciousness or fainting, as previously discussed. While syncope can occur occasionally in anyone and may not necessarily indicate a serious illness, it can sometimes lead to severe injuries. Additionally, syncope can serve as a warning sign preceding an episode of sudden cardiac arrest, leading to death within minutes.

There are two crucial causes of cardiac syncope: cardiac rhythm disorders (arrhythmias) and cardiomyopathy. The first, Hypertrophic Cardiomyopathy (HCM), involves cardiac muscle thickening. The arrhythmia can be tachyarrhythmia (fast heartbeat) like ventricular tachycardia, ventricular fibrillation, or Bradyarrhythmia (slow heartbeat), which includes sinus nodal disease and AV conduction disorder. Both conditions can lead to electrical problems, sudden collapse, and cardiac arrest. It is essential to differentiate between cardiac arrest, an electrical problem, and a heart attack, primarily a circulatory issue. Cardiac arrest is far more severe than a heart attack, as it involves a sudden, complete cessation of heart activity.

Prompt evaluation is crucial for the syncope as it can lead to cardiac arrest and sudden cardiac death. In some instances, heart attack patients may also develop arrhythmias leading to sudden cardiac arrest during their heart attack; they are those patients who die while shifting to a hospital or in transit. It further emphasizes the importance of swift medical attention in patients with chest pain followed by collapse.

Noncardiac but Vascular symptoms

Intermittent Claudication: In addition to the five critical cardiac complaints we discussed earlier—easy fatigability, syncope, palpitation, breathlessness, and chest pain—intermittent claudication is another symptom that can signal the presence of heart disease in the background of peripheral vascular disease (PVD). When someone experiences intermittent claudication, they feel catching pain in their calf muscle (leg) while walking, which subsides or disappears entirely upon resting. This condition is associated with an increased risk of developing heart disease. Data shows that approximately 50% of patients with intermittent claudication may have coronary blocks, although this issue is not directly related to the heart but to the circulatory vessels.

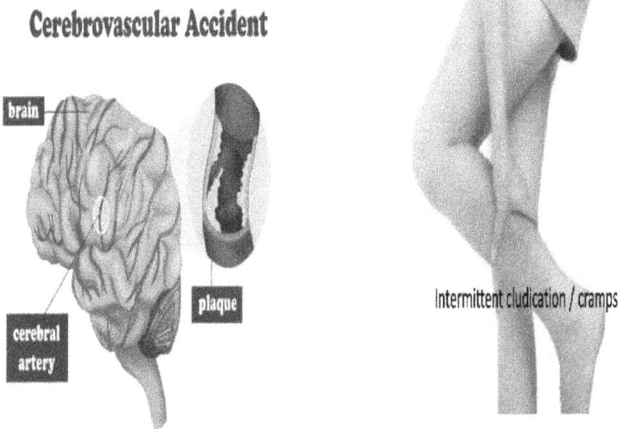

Cerebrovascular Accident

brain

cerebral artery

plaque

Intermittent cludication / cramps

Symptom of Peripheral Arterial Disease

Atherosclerosis is a cardiovascular disease characterized by blockages in blood vessels or arteries. Depending on the affected arteries, it can cause different organ-specific issues. For instance, blockages in brain arteries result in cerebral vascular disease, leading to brain strokes *(CVA)* or transient ischemic attacks *(TIA* -mini-strokes). On the other hand, blockages in the kidney's circulation cause renal vascular disease, potentially leading to kidney failure and hypertension. This type of hypertension is called secondary hypertension, where the cause is known and can be treated. If secondary hypertension is detected early, then interventions like stenting or opening the affected vessel to relieve hypertension can be performed. Unlike the more common primary hypertension with unknown causes, secondary hypertension can be managed and treated effectively once diagnosed.

Thus, the manifestations of cardiovascular diseases are diverse, affecting various organs outside the heart. They can lead to severe consequences, including brain strokes, kidney failure, and peripheral vascular disease, presenting with gangrene and needing amputation.

Early Detection of a Disease

Prevention is fundamental in medicine, and early detection is crucial for effective management. Family history plays a significant role in determining an individual's predisposition to certain diseases. Knowing the risk factors in one's family can help identify potential health issues and prompt early evaluation and prevention.

Non-infectious diseases such as diabetes, hypertension, coronary artery disease, and arrhythmias often have a strong genetic basis. If these conditions are present in the family history, evaluating whether the person has already developed any related conditions is essential. Early medical check-ups can help detect abnormalities and assess the individual's risk. An example of the importance of early detection is hypertrophic cardiomyopathy (HCM), a condition where the heart muscles become thick, leading to sudden cardiac events in athletes and young adults. Early evaluation becomes crucial if there is a family history of sudden deaths related to heart disease. Potential diseases can be diagnosed or ruled out with a few tests, and appropriate preventive measures can be taken.

Understanding **Gene Anticipation** is vital in diseases like hypertension, where the onset may occur earlier in subsequent generations. When the signs and symptoms of some genetic conditions tend to become more severe and appear earlier as the disorder is passed from generation to generation, it is called gene anticipation. Individuals with a family history of hypertension should not wait until the typical age of onset. Still, they should be proactive in managing their health from a younger age to prevent or delay the development of the condition. Awareness of family history and genetic implications can guide patients to make informed decisions about their health and take preventive actions.

Common Risk Factors for Heart Health

1. Smoking: Smoking is a well-known and harmful habit. It affects the smoker and poses risks to those exposed to second-hand smoke. The nicotine in tobacco is addictive and can cause oxidative injury to the inner lining of blood vessels, leading to endothelial inflammation and atherosclerosis. Passive smoking, inhaling smoke from others, can also increase the risk of heart-related diseases.

2. Air Pollution: High levels of air pollution, especially PM2.5 particles (2.5 micrometers or less in diameter), can also initiate endothelial dysfunction and inflammation, like smoking. Living in industrial areas or polluted cities can increase the risk of atherosclerosis.

3. Obesity: Obesity is a significant risk factor for heart disease and other health issues, including certain cancers. It can lead to vascular inflammation and increase the likelihood of atherosclerosis. BMI is one measure to identify obesity, but even individuals with normal BMI may have excess abdominal fat, contributing to inflammation.

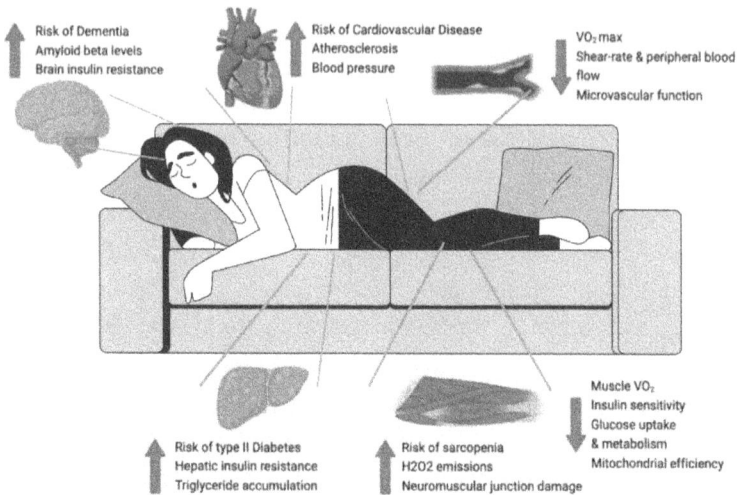

Risk of Dementia
Amyloid beta levels
Brain insulin resistance

Risk of Cardiovascular Disease
Atherosclerosis
Blood pressure

VO₂ max
Shear-rate & peripheral blood flow
Microvascular function

Risk of type II Diabetes
Hepatic insulin resistance
Triglyceride accumulation

Risk of sarcopenia
H2O2 emissions
Neuromuscular junction damage

Muscle VO₂
Insulin sensitivity
Glucose uptake
& metabolism
Mitochondrial efficiency

Sedentary lifestyle and Risks associated with it

4. Sedentary Lifestyle: Prolonged sitting without regular exercise has become a dangerous risk factor. Sitting for more than six hours daily without physical activity increases the risk of various diseases comparable to smoking. Sedentary behavior can negatively impact overall health and cardiovascular well-being.

I once treated a 22-year-old college guy with quite an unexpected health scare. One fine day, he was hit with intense chest pain, and when they checked his heart's electrical map (ECG), it was screaming "ACS" (that's short for ST-elevation Myocardial Infarction, a serious heart situation). But what's puzzling is that this young college kid seemed to have the odds in his favor. His cholesterol levels were on point, he didn't have diabetes or high blood pressure, he wasn't a smoker or a drinker, and even his family tree had no signs of early heart trouble. Sounds like a pretty healthy boy, right? This boy has a unique thing worth mentioning. He was on the heavier side with a BMI of 29 and sporting a bit of a belly. But the real twist was in his lifestyle. For the past three years, he'd been living the ultimate gamer's dream, practically glued to his room, gaming with friends online. Late-night junk food munching was a regular thing, and it was all about pizza, burgers, biryani, and plenty of sugary soft drinks. He'd stay up all hours, glued to his computer screen, with daily online classes.

Now, here's where things get serious. This lifestyle is like sending out an open invitation to trouble, even if you don't have the typical risk factors for heart issues. It led to clot formation in one of his major heart arteries. But don't worry, there's a happy ending to this story. He underwent a procedure called Thrombosuction, and he bounced back. I gave him valuable advice: Make significant changes in his lifestyle, starting with shedding some weight. So, this case reminds us that even if you don't have the usual suspects for heart problems, your lifestyle can still lead you down a rocky path. It's a lesson in caring for your heart, even if you're young and seemingly healthy.

5. Genetic - Present time epidemic of coronary artery disease, diabetes, dyslipidemia, some arrhythmia, and cardiomyopathy has polygenic and monogenic underpinning. While awareness about parameters like hemoglobin, sugar, and cholesterol levels is growing, the importance of genetics on heart health remains relatively overlooked in the public domain—individuals with a family history of diabetes, hypertension, or coronary artery disease. Early check-ups, proper follow-ups, and adhering to healthy lifestyle choices can help prevent the manifestation of genetic patterns. Moreover, promoting genetic testing and counseling can give individuals insights into their unique health risks, empowering them to take proactive measures toward better heart health. Knowledge of one's genetic predispositions can lead to tailored preventive strategies, including lifestyle modifications and early detection of potential issues.

6. **Alcohol consumption** has been the subject of much research and debate regarding its effects on heart health. Some observational studies have suggested that moderate alcohol intake, particularly in the form of wine, may benefit heart health due to the presence of *Resveratrol*, an antioxidant and anti-inflammatory compound found in red wine. However, it's important to note that these studies are <u>observational</u> and not randomized controlled trials, which means the evidence is not for cause-and-effect establishment called causal

association. There are a lot of confounding factors which bias the observation studies. Alcohol, in general, is habit-forming and inflammatory for mitochondria, which are essential parts of our cells responsible for energy production. Therefore, regular and excessive alcohol consumption can harm overall health, including the cardiovascular system. While moderate alcohol intake may not have significant adverse effects for some individuals, it is crucial to be cautious as it can still lead to habit formation and other potential health risks.

For individuals with certain heart conditions like PSVT (Paroxysmal Supraventricular Tachycardia), caffeinated drinks (tea, coffee, or chocolate) can trigger episodes of the condition. Similarly, alcohol consumption, particularly binge drinking, may also increase the risk of Atrial fibrillation recurrence in such cases. Therefore, people with heart conditions must know these triggers and make necessary lifestyle adjustments to avoid potential complications.

The upper limit of alcohol consumption to avoid liver diseases is generally defined as less than two drinks per day for males and less than one drink per day for females. However, individuals with hypertension, diabetes, or Coronary Artery Disease (CAD) are often advised to avoid alcohol, as it can exacerbate these conditions and increase the risk of other cardiovascular issues, such as atrial fibrillation.

Binge drinking should be strictly avoided, as it can harm the heart, including an increased risk of atrial fibrillation, a rhythm disorder leading to a higher risk of stroke. Social drinking in moderation may be more tolerable for some individuals, but it's still essential to consider individual health conditions and hazards.

There are some studies suggesting the potential benefits of moderate alcohol intake. However, the evidence is not conclusive, and alcohol consumption should be approached with caution, especially for individuals with existing heart conditions or other health risk factors. It's essential to consult with healthcare professionals to understand how alcohol consumption may affect one's specific health condition and overall well-being.

Food Habits

1. Junk Food and Processed Foods: Consuming junk food and heavily processed foods is detrimental to heart health. These foods often contain high levels of trans fatty acids and lack essential nutrients, leading to poor heart function.

2. Irregular Eating Habits: Eating irregularly and incredibly late at night can disrupt natural digestion and affect the gut microbiota. This disturbance in the gut can lead to various health issues, including heart disease, cancer, depression, and stroke.

3. Timing of Food Intake: Eating your food during the daytime will be more in line with our natural rhythms. But if you practice eating at night, especially with the increasing trend of midnight food delivery services, it can lead to health problems as it violates nature's patterns.

Individuals must be aware of these risk factors and consciously adopt a healthy lifestyle. Avoiding smoking and exposure to pollution, maintaining a healthy weight, engaging in regular physical activity, and following balanced and timely eating habits are essential for preserving heart health and overall well-being. Awareness and preventive measures can significantly reduce the risk of heart-related diseases and other health issues.

3

CARDIAC INVESTIGATIONS & DIAGNOSIS

"Small is the number of them that see with their own eyes and feel with their own hearts."

— **Albert Einstein**

Upon reaching a medical facility or hospital, the first crucial step is to conduct thorough medical investigations to accurately detect and diagnose the underlying disease before initiating appropriate treatment. Due to the compact arrangement of our bodily organs, symptoms of different diseases can often overlap, making it challenging to distinguish between them. Hence, precise diagnosis is paramount to ensure effective treatment, especially regarding heart-related conditions, as misdiagnoses can have life-threatening consequences.

Diagnosing a heart disease

In today's world, medical practitioners have abundant resources, including advanced diagnostic equipment, to aid in disease diagnosis. But to an extent, the clinical skills of doctors have diminished over time due to the reliance on technology. Modern medicine often tends to be diagnosis-based, with practitioners immediately resorting to diagnostic tools for confirmation.

In the past, experienced medical practitioners relied on their investigative skills to understand the patient's complaints thoroughly and conduct careful evaluations before arriving at a diagnosis. They would consider the timing and pattern of symptoms and analyze the patient's medical history and risk factors. Such practitioners would be up-to-date with medical knowledge and keenly observe the patient's response to initial treatments.

Contrastingly, the modern approach involves ordering tests without adequately listening to the patient or understanding the disease. Excessive reliance on tests can lead to confusing borderline diagnoses, and patients may be referred to multiple specialists.

In conclusion, maintaining a balance between modern diagnostic tools and the skills of experienced medical practitioners is crucial for accurate and comprehensive disease diagnosis. Listening to patients, understanding their complaints, and conducting thorough investigations can lead to a more wholesome diagnosis, reducing unnecessary tests and costs while providing optimal patient care.

Basic Investigations Through Blood Tests

With the advancements in modern medical technology, we now have a plethora of non-invasive and invasive investigations available to diagnose various heart conditions. However, the initial step in any medical investigation usually begins with a basic blood test, which is non-invasive. A small blood sample can provide essential insights into your health, including comorbidities or illnesses. For instance, low hemoglobin levels can cause various issues as hemoglobin is a crucial protein inside red blood cells responsible for carrying oxygen throughout the body. It is vital to ensure sufficient hemoglobin levels to facilitate efficient oxygen delivery to all body parts. Correcting low hemoglobin is a priority before addressing any other cardiac ailments, as it may be the root cause that needs immediate attention.

- Fasting glucose>126 mg/dl (7 mmol/l)
  or
- Post prandial glucose>200 mg/dl (11.1 mmol/l)
  or
- HbA1c>6.5%(48 mmol/mol)
  and
- Insulin deficiency
- Clinical signs of an insulin deficiency syndrom (polyuria, polydipsie, weightloss, ketoacidosis)

The Total Leukocyte Count (TLC) and Differential Leukocyte Count (DLC) are assessed following hemoglobin analysis. Leukocytes, or white blood cells, play a crucial role in the immune system, protecting the body against infections. Low TLC and DLC levels indicate a higher susceptibility to infections and can provide clues about inflammatory conditions.

The following important test is the fasting and postprandial blood sugar. The hemoglobin A1c (HbA1c) test provides valuable information about your sugar levels over the past three months, helping determine your diabetes and evaluate your diabetic profile. A fasting level of 126mg/dl or above or postprandial sugar of more than 200mg/dl is the standard definition of diabetes, provided it is done in 10 hours of fasting, and the person is not in acute illness. Diabetes is the mother of all diseases. None of the body's organ system is spared, and it affects the function of *all organs*. Hence, good blood sugar control is vital in preventing heart disease and its complications. A primary risk factor for heart ailments, making this test particularly relevant in assessing heart-related illnesses.

Furthermore, serum creatinine, urea, sodium, and potassium levels, which are parameters related to kidney function, are measured. Creatinine is a waste product that kidneys filter from the blood and excrete through urine. Elevated creatinine levels in the blood can be a warning sign for kidney issues. When analyzing their creatinine levels, it is essential to consider a patient's age, as this parameter is age-dependent and influenced by muscle mass. Kidney function is crucial for metabolizing and excreting many medications, including cardiac drugs. It is essential to tailor drug choice and dosage based on a patient's kidney function, especially for long-term cardiac medication use.

Continuing with the investigations, monitoring Sodium and Potassium levels is also crucial, as some medications may raise these levels. Elevated potassium can lead to electrical conduction abnormalities in the heart's muscle tissue, including complete heart block. Close monitoring and careful dosage titration are necessary for certain patients to maintain appropriate levels. Low Sodium levels indicate fluid accumulation in the body, leading to a decrease in sodium levels. It is an indirect indicator that the dosage needs adjustment to reduce water retention and ease the strain on the heart. Urea or uric acid levels indirectly reflect the kidneys' fluid status, metabolism rate, and absorbent status.

Elevated levels of these liver enzymes in the blood can signal inflammation and damage to liver cells. In certain heart-related diseases, there can be a backflow effect on the lungs and liver, leading to liver congestion or infarcts, causing these enzyme counts to surpass 1000. In such cases, toxic drugs must be avoided, and medicines to relieve liver congestion and support heart function are prescribed.

The blood's total albumin and protein levels are also critical liver-related parameters. Albumin, produced by the liver, comprises a significant portion of the blood's protein. Low albumin levels can lead to water retention in the body. If combined with reduced heart pumping, liver decongestion becomes difficult even with medications, as many drugs rely on albumin or protein for transport and effectiveness. Thus, albumin levels are crucial in determining drug dosage and treatment plans.

These basic minimum tests help investigate diseases and design personalized treatment methods based on different blood parameters. Monitoring and understanding these essential factors are vital for accurate diagnosis and effective treatment of heart and other related diseases.

Lipid Profiling

After considering the basic parameters, the lipid profile provides essential clues underlying the risk of developing heart disease. In the lipid profile, LDL (Low-Density Lipoprotein) and HDL (High-Density Lipoprotein) are crucial parameters. However, a unique lipoprotein known as Lipoprotein(a) or Lp(a) has been identified as a risk factor and marker for atherosclerosis or vascular diseases. Patients with Lp(a) levels above 30mg/dl may be genetically predisposed to heart diseases at an early age, and there might also be a family history of such conditions. This association is also linked to Homocysteine (Hcy), a naturally produced non-proteinogenic α-amino acid in our body. Elevated Homocysteine levels indicate increased blood thickness, leading to a higher risk of coagulation and clot formation associated with various diseases. Another serum biomarker, High-sensitivity C-reactive protein (hsCRP), produced by the liver, indicates the presence of inflammation in the body. These biomarkers are used for selected patients to assess the severity of inflammation but are not the primary targets for treatment. They provide valuable information about inflammation levels and its impact on the body.

Next, a complete urine examination is essential to detect ongoing infections and determine if urine is losing protein. The urine albumin-creatinine ratio (UACR) measures the amount of albumin kidneys are losing, and values up to 30 milligrams/gm daily are considered normal. However, levels above 30 milligrams/gm, up to 300 milligrams (microalbuminuria), and more than 300 milligrams/gm (macroalbuminuria) indicate endothelial dysfunction and an increased risk of cardiovascular ailments. Even non-diabetic patients with abnormal UACR levels face a higher risk of developing heart attack or hypertension. Protein loss marks a critical turning point in a person's health trajectory, potentially leading to kidney disease and, eventually, heart ailments. Treating patients based on their specific stage is essential to slow undesirable disease progression.

These blood markers and tests form the foundation of most basic non-invasive investigations conducted for patients, including routine health check-ups. The valuable insights gained from these tests help healthcare professionals diagnose diseases accurately and design appropriate treatment plans for each individual.

Acute or Critical Emergencies

When a patient arrives at the hospital in an acute emergency, three critical blood markers (**myocardial injury markers**) are immediately tested to diagnose a cardiac illness, especially when the exact onset of chest pain is unknown. These markers are Trop T (Troponin T), Trop I (Troponin I), and CPK-MB (Creatine Phosphokinase Myocardial Band). Even a slight elevation in troponin or CK-MB levels indicates a heart illness, and if the levels are higher, it suggests a heart attack may have occurred within the last 48 hours. CPK-MB is elevated during the first 48 hours of a heart attack, while Trop T and Trop I remain elevated for 10 to 14 days. The rising trend is the mark of heart injury. These tests help determine the time since the attack occurred, aiding in the diagnosis and selection of appropriate treatment, as discussed in earlier chapters.

The **ECG** provides crucial information about the acuteness of the emergency. It helps detect ST elevation MI, which indicates a blocked coronary artery and the need for thrombolysis or primary angioplasty to address heart attacks with compromised circulation. The ECG also assesses the electrical flow in the heart and can identify rhythm disorders, electrolyte imbalances, and possible conditions like dilated or hypertrophic chambers. While the ECG offers definitive information about a heart attack, it may not always be sensitive enough for all other findings. However, changes in the ST elevation, ST depression, and ST wave inversion segments can be observed on the ECG. This allows conclusions about the type and severity of heart disease, the presence of blockages, and whether a heart attack is ongoing or old. ECG also provides information regarding the electrical flow of current. The normal electrical flow that happens from the upper chambers and comes to the lower chamber can be nicely traced by ECG. Any current electrical block between the upper and lower chambers is called an AV block. There are three degrees in severity -first degree, second degree, and the most severe, called third degree when no current flows from the upper chamber to the lower chamber (also called a complete heart block). ECG also provides the conduction state of the right and left bundle of conduction. The slowing of conduction in the right and left bundle branches is called *the right and left bundle branch block*, but it **is "not block,"** but the speed of conduction in those bundles is destined to provide current to the lower chamber(ventricle).

Holter recorders are used for prolonged ECG monitoring for patients experiencing intermittent symptoms of palpitation. This allows for detecting abnormal heart rates or rhythms and aids in diagnosing arrhythmia. **Loop recorder**s are similar to Holter, and they record for a longer duration of up to 2 weeks. They can be external loop recorders and implantable loop recorders (ILR). ILR can record the ECG in real time for three years. Nowadays, we have patch ECG, comprised of a small patch attached to the chest and connected to a mobile with Bluetooth. The ECG recording in this system is real-time.

A non-invasive method called **TMT (Treadmill Test)** is used for patients with suspected coronary artery disease that falls in an intermediate risk category. During a TMT, the patient walks or runs on a treadmill while their heart rate and ECG are monitored. The stress gradually increases, and heart rate and ECG changes are observed. TMT provides indirect clues about the behavior of heart circulation and helps assess whether the patient has coronary artery blockages. The appearance of specific ECG changes during the

TMT, such as ST depressions, ST elevations, VT or VF, or hypotensive rhythm, indicates a severely compromised cardiovascular condition.

TMT is recommended for patients who do not exhibit apparent ECG abnormalities in their resting state. Controlled stress on a treadmill can reveal essential clues on the ECG, aiding in risk assessment, evaluation, and treatment planning for the patient.

The combination of blood marker tests and ECG provides critical diagnostic information to guide immediate and appropriate treatment for patients experiencing cardiac emergencies.

Echocardiography remains a valuable tool for assessing heart pumping function valve performance, and detecting structural heart diseases (chambers dimension). Echocardiography, also known as an Echo test/ 2D echo, is a vital investigation that provides two crucial details about the heart: its pumping function and the status of valves & chambers. This non-invasive test is critical in newborn babies to assess whether the heart is typical or if there are any congenital heart conditions. The Echo test can clearly show the presence of holes in the heart, known as shunts, indicating abnormal connections between the left and right chambers. It is the most reliable investigative tool for evaluating chamber anatomy, size, and positioning. Echocardiography also offers a detailed view of all four valves in the heart: the mitral, tricuspid, aortic, and pulmonary valves. This allows for a comprehensive assessment of valve function and muscle performance, enabling the identification of any structural congenital heart disease or valvular heart disease.

Moreover, in cases of ongoing heart attacks or symptoms suggesting a heart attack, Echocardiography can provide additional information based on the expertise of the interpreting physician. Experienced cardiac experts can analyze the type of contraction observed in the Echo to pinpoint the specific territory of the heart that may not be moving correctly. While the exact timeline of the heart attack cannot be determined with certainty, particular characteristics observed in the Echo, such as thinning or contraction patterns, can offer clues about the timing and the particular coronary artery that may be blocked or compromised. This information is especially relevant in evaluation cases of coronary artery disease (CAD).

Echocardiography is an invaluable investigation for assessing heart function, chamber anatomy, valve function, and the presence of structural or valvular heart diseases. Echocardiography can accurately define and diagnose cases where blood accumulates around the heart chambers due to pericardial issues or pericarditis. However, it is essential to note that Echocardiography is not a definitive diagnostic tool for detecting coronary blocks in patients in asymptomatic conditions. It can provide clues if an ongoing heart attack corroborates with ECG findings but may not provide information about coronary flow or block in it. The **transesophageal Echocardiogram (TEE)** is a procedure in which an Echocardiography probe is mounted on the endoscope and through the food pipe(esophagus) passed in the lower esophagus and stomach to visualize the heart from the back side(posterior side). It became beneficial when the hole was suspected at the upper chamber level(ASD) or suspected internal tear in the Aorta(dissection of the Aorta). **Dobutamine stress Echocardiogram(DSE)** provides information similar to TMT. This is conducted when the patient cannot walk fast or run due to physical disability. It gives a clue if any coronary circulation is compromised or not.

Moving to the next level of investigations, CT Angiography and Coronary Angiography play significant roles. **CT Angiography,** performed in the radiology department, involves introducing a contrast dye into a peripheral vein to visualize the heart and its vessels inside. This provides valuable information about the heart chamber's blood flow and can *rule out three critical emergencies*: coronary blockage, aortic dissection, and pulmonary embolism. Additionally, CT Angiography can be used in selected patients for coronary assessment on an outpatient basis. Sometimes, it may supplement a routine coronary angiogram to visualize better coronary ostia (the opening of coronary arteries) and the anomalous course of coronary arteries. However, it is essential to note that CT Angiography may have limitations in visualizing the distal parts of the coronary arteries or narrow arteries, and the quality of the images can vary based on the type of CT scan performed (16 slices, 64 slices, 132 slices).

Coronary artery Calcium(CAC) Scan is another diagnostic tool that utilizes a CT Scan to measure the amount of calcium in the coronary artery, a mark of atherosclerosis in the calcified stage. Coronary artery calcium (CAC) scan is a simple, proven test for detecting and quantifying calcific coronary atherosclerosis. Calcium has been associated with coronary artery disease (CAD) and heart blocks. Calcium Scoring is primarily used as a screening tool for coronary artery disease in patients with risk factors and asymptomatic. If the calcium Screening indicates a high calcium level (>400HU), further investigation with coronary angiography can be performed to visualize the blockages more closely and plan the appropriate treatment. A zero score is always taken bad in real life, but in a CAC scan, it is considered best from a CAD point of view, but there is a fallacy. CAC testing has been unable to detect and quantify noncalcified coronary atherosclerotic plaque, plaque features, or lumen stenosis, which are responsible for most heart attacks (ACS), hence missing the elephant. Secondly, for patients younger than 40 years., CAC is not adding risk assessment and, most of the time, zero as the CAD has not entered the calcific atherosclerotic phase. Hence, a zero score in CAC in young patients provides a false sense of complacency to the person. CAC testing is not recommended for symptomatic patients where a CT angiogram or routine coronary angiogram is an investigation of choice.

Coronary Angiography, an invasive procedure, involves inserting catheters near the coronary arteries and injecting a dye for video contrast to visualize the blockages in detail. This procedure allows for a clear assessment of the blockage's number, location, and severity. Based on the results of the Angiogram, the next level of treatment can be planned, which could include angioplasty with stenting or open-heart bypass surgery in some cases. Coronary

Angiography is typically performed as a day procedure in the cardiology department.

Cardiac Catheterization study, also called "**Cath study**," is done in selected patients with heart failure, congenital heart disease, and cardiac transplant pulmonary artery hypertension to identify various parameters essential in clinical decision-making. It involves real-time pressure measurement in cardiac chambers and great vessels. It involves sampling blood oxygenation levels at different chambers to identify blood mixing in complex congenital heart diseases with holes(shunt). It is also done to determine whether the patient is suitable for cardiac transplant and to know the immune system's response to a transplanted heart.

Radionuclide Scanning is another valuable imaging technique used in cardiovascular diagnosis. Radionuclide imaging uses a special detector (gamma camera) to create an image following the injection of radioactive material. Radionuclide imaging can expose patients to similar amounts of radiation than comparable computed tomography (CT) studies. However, because the patient briefly retains the radioactive material, sophisticated radiation alarms (e.g., in airports) may be triggered by the patient for several days after such testing. It involves using a small amount of a radioactive isotope Radioactive thallium-201 (Tl-201), Technetium-99m (Tc-99m) markers (sestamibi, tetrofosmin, and teboroxime)as a tracer to observe the heart's muscles, (myocardium) perfusion, valvular function, and pumping, with compromised coronary circulation. It determines whether revascularization in the particular coronary territory with stenting or bypass surgery will be a fruitful means of improving myocardial contractility, thus providing the functional impact of the block. Tc-99m pyrophosphate is used similarly to evaluate cardiac involvement in transthyretin amyloidosis (a type of amyloidosis in which sheets of misfolded transthyretin protein can accumulate in tissues, including the heart). It runs in familial disease.

Cardiac MRI (Magnetic Resonance Imaging) is an advanced diagnostic tool that provides comprehensive information that complements the information of Echocardiography but with additional details and adds information about the viability of and inflammation of heart muscle. Cardiac MRI offers insights into muscle behavior during contraction, perfusion levels, and the presence of any scars. This is a *destination investigation* in evaluating heart myocardial, valvular, and coronary as any structural abnormality or disease. It is a taking procedure, and claustrophobia in patients can be restricted in some patients. The presence of an abandoned pacemaker or ICD lead is a contraindication to undergo MRI.

PET (Positron Emission Tomography) scan checks for inflammation, which can affect various bodily organs, including the heart. A PET scan can be performed when inflammation specifically affects the heart and other organs are clear of it. During this scan, a radioisotope tracer called FDG (Fluorodeoxyglucose) is given, accumulating at the inflamed region as they need more glucose in normal tissue, allowing visualization of the FDG uptake. Targeting the inflamed region can initiate targeted treatment with medications or devices. PET scan is also used to investigate diseases unrelated to the heart, but in this context, it is utilized to detect inflammation within the heart.

These diagnostic investigations play a crucial role in managing cardiovascular disease, whether acute or chronic. Medical professionals consider the patient's overall health and condition while determining the most appropriate diagnostic approach for individual cases. The random packages for health evaluation either by diagnostic center or hospital is not a holistic approach or cost-effective most of the time.

4

DIET FOR HEALTH

"Only one-fourth of our food makes us live, remaining makes the doctor live."

-Egyptian Proverb

To perform all physical and mental activities, we need nutrition, which is the essential component of the food. In the early stages of human civilization, our primitive ancestors relied on their instincts and ate only when they experienced hunger pangs. Survival was their primary focus, much like that of other animals in the wild. As time progressed, humans transitioned from hunting for food during the day to cultivating and cooking food, leading to changes in their eating habits.

Today, however, our food habits have evolved significantly, and it's essential to examine how we consume food in the modern era. There is an African proverb for this scenario: "1/4 of what you eat keeps you alive, and 3/4 keeps your doctor alive." This proverb aptly emphasizes that only a quarter of our food is necessary for survival and sustenance. At the same time, the rest contribute to various illnesses, making overconsumption a prevalent issue in this era. As a result, numerous complex diseases have emerged due to our excessive and unhealthy eating habits.

We are what we eat, and in ancient times, people faced primarily infectious diseases that they combated with natural immunity. Natural immunity depends on genetics, food choices, and lifestyle. Our ancestors gathered food from the wild jungles. The food was natural and abundant, and they did physical labor throughout the day. So they had robust immune systems. However, the advent of inventions like electricity and cooking gas brought significant changes, leading to a shift in eating patterns.

There is a surplus of food in the modern era, offering various foods throughout the year and even globally. However, this abundance has resulted in a disparity in food consumption levels, leading to malnutrition in some regions and overconsumption in others. Diseases like Diabetes, Hypertension, Coronary Artery Disease (CAD), and some cancers are directly related to excessive food intake and its effect on obesity.

Living far from nature and urbanization has led us to detach from the natural environment, affecting our immune systems negatively. By limiting our interactions with nature, we compromise our immune defenses and pass on these vulnerabilities to future generations through genetics. Additionally, autoimmune diseases, where the immune system attacks the body's cells, have become more prevalent due to these changes. While the heart has largely been spared from autoimmune diseases, new complexities and challenges arise in maintaining overall health. Returning to a more natural and balanced way of living is crucial to preserving and enhancing heart health. Adopting healthier eating habits, consuming foods in moderation, and staying physically active are essential steps toward preventing heart diseases and maintaining overall well-being. By reconnecting with nature and adopting healthier lifestyles, we can strengthen our immune systems and protect ourselves from the burdens of modern diseases. In our pursuit of good health, three essential components demand our attention when it comes to food: the *timing* of consumption, the *quality* of what we eat, and the *quantity* of our food intake. These aspects profoundly impact our overall well-being and are vital to our nutrition and health.

Timing of Food

Throughout history, humans have been eating naturally, consuming food during the daytime and resting at night. However, with modern advancements like electricity, technology, and the convenience of home delivery, we have deviated from this natural rhythm. The availability of food 24x7, combined with round-the-clock entertainment, has led to irregular eating habits, disconnecting us from our natural way of nourishment. "when we eat is as

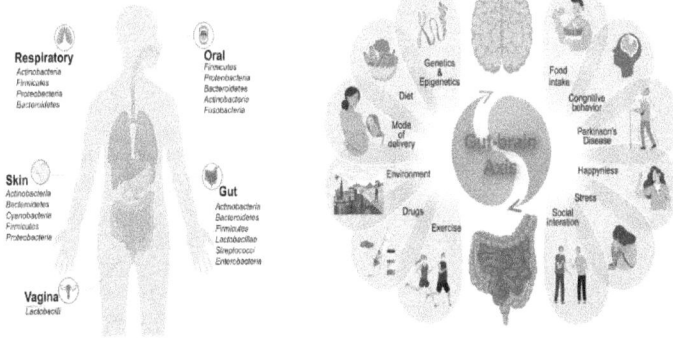

Microbiota composition in different regions

Respiratory
Actinobacteria
Firmicutes
Proteobacteria
Bacteroidetes

Oral
Firmicutes
Proteobacteria
Bacteroidetes
Actinobacteria
Fusobacteria

Skin
Actinobacteria
Bacteroidetes
Cyanobacteria
Firmicutes
Proteobacteria

Gut
Actinobacteria
Bacteroidetes
Firmicutes
Lactobacillae
Streptococci
Enterobacteria

Vagina
Lactobacilli

Genetics & Epigenetics
Diet
Mode of delivery
Environment
Drugs
Exercise
Gut-brain Axis
Food Intake
Cognitive behavior
Parkinson's Disease
Happyniess
Stress
Social Interaction

Microbiota composition in different regions-Gut-brain Axis

important as what we eat."

This disruption also affects our gut microbiota, a collection of microorganisms in our intestines. These microbiotas are crucial in digestion and nutrient absorption and support our immune system. Irregular eating patterns can disturb this delicate balance, potentially leading to various health issues, including cancers, heart diseases, and depression.

Giving our microbiota ample time to rest and adapt to our food is vital. Constantly bombarding them with food at odd hours can lead to mutations and malfunctions, contributing to autoimmune diseases and other health problems. Research has shown that time-restricted eating can have significant health benefits when we adhere to specific eating windows during the day. In a study on mice by Dr. Satchidananda Panda, mice who ate within a set amount of time (8-12 hours) resulted in slimmer, healthier mice than those who ate the same number of calories in a larger window of time, showing that when one eats may be as important as what one eats.

By embracing disciplined eating habits, ideally between sunrise and sunset, as was customary in ancient times, we can reduce the risk of many diseases and improve our overall health. Confining caloric consumption to an 8- to 12-hour period—as people did just a century ago—might stave off high cholesterol, diabetes, and obesity.

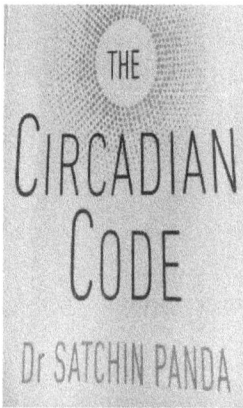

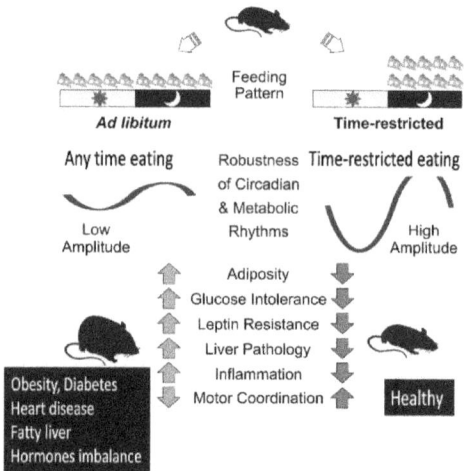

The Microbiota

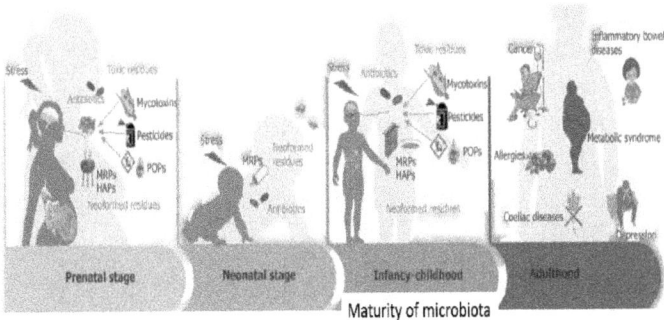

Maturity of microbiota

It was found that many microorganisms, including bacteria, yeasts, and viruses, coexist in various human body sites (gut, skin, lung, and oral cavity). In addition, the human microbiota, also known as "the hidden organ," contributes over 150 times more genetic information than the entire human genome. Unsurprisingly, the gut microbiota, considered the largest endocrine organ in the body, can affect the cardiovascular system and contribute to CVDs. Gut microbiota is regarded as the most significant one in maintaining our health. Intestinal microbial balance is closely relevant to human diseases and health. Compared with other body regions, the human gastrointestinal (GI) tract contains an abundant microbial community that gathers ~100 trillion microorganisms. The gut microbiota exhibits stability, resilience, and symbiotic interaction with the host in healthy conditions. At about age 3, children's gut microbiota becomes comparable to that of adults. Generally, the microbiota diversity increases between childhood and adulthood and decreases at older age (over 70).

Gut microbiota was identified as a critical gut-brain axis regulator. A study that transplanted the microbiota from Parkinson's disease patients to mice showed enhanced physical impairments compared with mice with microbiota from healthy donors.

Thus, it suggests that gut microbes are potentially relevant to neurodegenerative diseases such as Parkinson's and could be used as a therapeutic marker.

Mounting evidence has confirmed that microbiota is associated with developing CVDs, cancer, respiratory diseases, diabetes, IBD, brain disorders, chronic kidney diseases, and liver diseases. While the general risk factors include atherosclerosis, hypertension, obesity, diabetes, dyslipidemia, and mental illness, growing evidence has suggested that microbiota play a role in maintaining cardiovascular health, and its dysregulation may contribute to CVDs If we make changes in the food type, timing, and overall environment; the microbiota will adapt which will potentially lead to disease-prone conditions. Gut microbiota is involved in choline, phosphatidylcholine, and carnitine metabolism, eventually producing trimethylamine-N-oxide (TMAO). TMAO has been suggested to regulate cholesterol balance and bile acid levels and is associated with early atherosclerosis and a high long-term mortality risk of CVDs. Increased fiber intake(polysaccharides) is associated with more SCFA (short-chain fatty acid) production by gut microbiota, including acetates, butyrates, or propionates. The butyrates mediate the integrity of the intestinal barrier and are suggested to have direct beneficial effects on intestinal epithelial cells. The propionates and butyrates protect the host from hypertensive cardiovascular damage.

Butyrate has a robust anti-inflammatory potential and constitutes the primary energy source for gut epithelial cells. At the same time, SCFA may be partly responsible for the benefits derived from consuming the fiber-rich Mediterranean diet. An elevated *Firmicutes/Bacteroidetes* ratio has been identified as a possible biomarker of gut dysbiosis and various diseases, such as T2DM, obesity, and coronary artery atherosclerotic heart disease. Most bacteria belonging to the phylum *Firmicutes* feature a gram-positive cell wall structure. They are associated with unhealthy lifestyles, such as a high-fat diet, abnormal energy balance, and being overweight. The story of Gut dysbiosis does not stop here. A recent study published in an esteemed journal circulation on July 2023 by a group

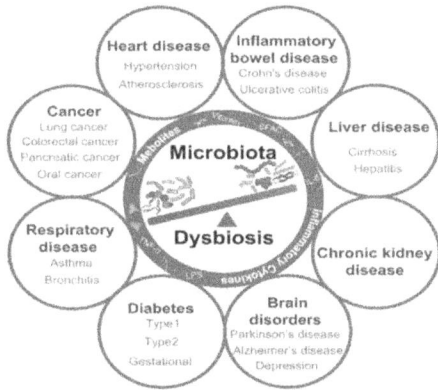

Microbiota Imbalance(dysbiosis) And Evolution Of Diseases

of scientists from Spain found Bacterial species common in the oral cavity, streptococci, most strongly correlating with Coronary Artery Calcium (CAC) scores, that is, *S anginosus*, *S oralis* subspecies *oralis*, and *S parasanguinis*. These bacteria may "contribute to atherogenesis by direct infection or by altering host metabolism which resides in as oral microbiota.

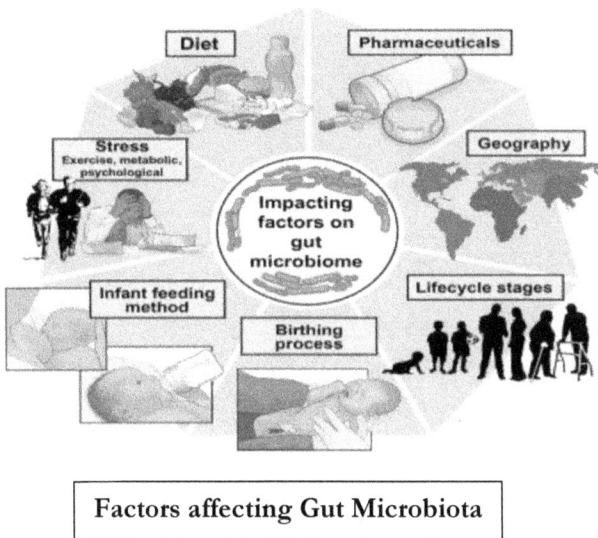

Factors affecting Gut Microbiota

Disciplining our eating timings can optimize the functioning of our gut microbiota, maintain a balanced immune response, and safeguard our overall health. Time-restricted eating allows our gut microbiota to perform efficiently, benefiting our digestion and immune system.

In conclusion, paying attention to the timing of our food intake and adopting a more natural and disciplined approach can promote better gut health, bolster immunity, and reduce the risk of chronic diseases. Embracing the practices of our ancestors by consuming food during the daytime and allowing our bodies to rest at night can foster overall well-being and contribute to a healthier life.

Quality of Food

Substantial evidence from a health and nature perspective supports the idea that vegetarian food is generally better for our well-being. Our dental structure, with more molar teeth and fewer pointed canine teeth, points to our inclination towards an herbivorous diet. Additionally, our long intestine, around 6.5 meters in length, favors the digestion of plant-based foods, which are high in cellulose and require more time for breakdown.

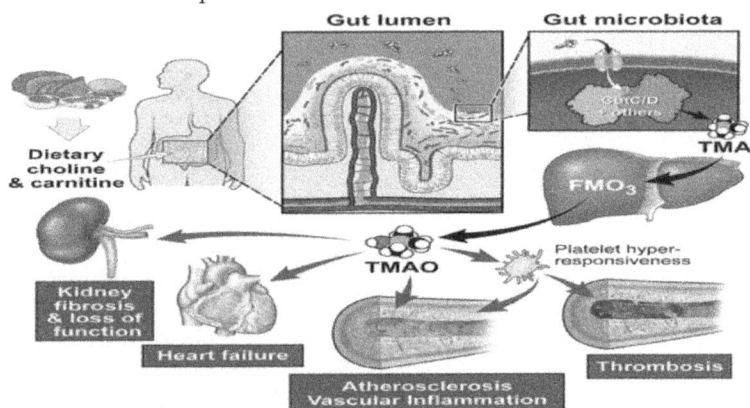

Vegetarian vs. Non-Vegetarian Food

While humans can consume meat in dire circumstances, our digestive system is better suited for a predominantly vegetarian diet. Studies have shown that excessive consumption of non-vegetarian food, particularly red meat, can lead to the release of Trimethylamine N-oxide (TMAO) in the blood, which activates vascular inflammation by activating the mitogen-activated protein kinase (MAPK) and NF-κB signaling pathways which are associated with inflammation and cancer cell proliferation. They are related to endothelial cells and smooth muscle cell proliferation and dysfunction that ultimately leads to the progression of atherosclerosis. TMAO has been associated with cholesterol metabolism adversely and is related to early atherosclerosis and a high long-term mortality risk of CVD. High non-vegetarian diets have also been associated with an increased risk of specific cancers (colorectal, breast, and prostate carcinoma).

The health benefits of dairy products depend on individual tolerances and dietary habits developed over time. Dairy may benefit some, while others might experience allergies or adverse effects.

Dangers of Pristine White

White symbolizes purity and innocence, but it is not so in the kitchen. Many food products with a pristine white appearance, such as sugar, salt, and white rice, can cause health-related problems if not restricted in quantity.

Sugar is considered one of the biggest enemies of human health, and its overconsumption has been linked to various health issues. Sugar is noteworthy as a substance that releases opioids and dopamine and has addictive potential. The neural adaptations include changes in dopamine and opioid receptor binding, enkephalin mRNA expression, and dopamine and acetylcholine release in the nucleus accumbens (the pleasure center). This reward and reinforcing effect translate into emotional stimulus and craving. Unsurprisingly, people get addicted to soft drinks, tea, coffee, and sugary products. Why can you not hold yourself after taking the first

Candy to the next Candy or the first drink to the next drink? The amalgamation of dopamine and opioids is most dangerous and has the potential for the addictive habit of any enriched sugary product.

This eating behavior does not happen when taking apples, bananas, or mangoes. While natural alternatives like jaggery are healthier, refined sugar undergoes extensive processing, losing valuable micronutrients and becoming a calorie-dense substance devoid of other essential nutrients.

Unlike natural foods that combine sugars, fibers, minerals, and vitamins, refined sugar only offers empty calories, leading to addiction due to the brain's response to increased sugar levels. This sugar addiction is dangerous and can contribute to various health problems, making it a *silent poison* that affects us over time.

Moving on from sugar, the next culprit in the kitchen is "common salt." In the past, people used rock salt, which contained enriching minerals and micronutrients like potassium, magnesium, and sometimes calcium. In contrast, although iodized, the powdered common salt commonly used today lacks these essential minerals. Sodium, present in common salt, can cause various health problems, but these can be balanced with the potassium, magnesium, and calcium in rock salt. Therefore, slightly discolored rock salt is a healthier alternative to pure white common salt.

The third white culprit in our kitchens is white rice, especially the polished white rice lacking the nutrient-rich layer under the husk. The nutrient layer contains essential nutrients like Vitamin B1 (Thiamin), which are necessary for preventing diseases like Beriberi. Unfortunately, much of the population relies solely on polished white rice without supplementation, leading to nutrient deficiencies and related health issues. Moreover, modern genetic engineering to produce hybrid rice may further compromise natural rice's quality and healthy enrichment.

Cooking oil

Next, let's discuss **cooking oil**. At the same time, some

observational studies have concluded that Mediterranean food and olive oil are beneficial for health due to their polyphenol content. However, olive oil might not be ideal for Indian cooking, which involves a lot of frying. Olive oil has a low rancidity threshold, making it less suitable for high-temperature frying.

On the other hand, **traditional ghee** is a rancidity-proof oil full of medium and short-chain fatty acids, including butyrates, which support a strong digestion, bile flow, and a healthy microbiome. Research suggests it can even shut off gene expression for cancer and inflammation. Contrary to popular belief, ghee does not raise cholesterol and is high in CLA (conjugated linoleic acid), which is needed to build lean muscle mass and support weight loss. It is a good source of fat-soluble vitamins, including A, D, E, and K. Ghee has been revered and used for various purposes, including worship, due to its high-quality properties and high smoke point (482 F), which makes it great for cooking.

In conclusion, opting for brown jaggery instead of refined white sugar, using slightly discolored rock salt over pure white common salt, and choosing natural rice with its nutrient-rich layer intact can significantly enhance the nutritional quality of our diet. Additionally, considering traditional ghee as a healthy cooking oil can be a wise choice for our overall well-being. Embracing these changes in our food habits can contribute to a healthier and more nourished life.

Ghee is the top choice for cooking oil if affordability is not an issue. However, when comparing other cooking oils with ghee, doubts often arise about which is better. Traditional cooking oils like mustard and groundnut oil surpass other options. The stickiness of an oil indicates its health benefits. Modern techniques used to refine or filter oils may compromise the quality and health properties of natural vegetable oils, notably after the refinement process, which includes chemical solvents, very high heat, and more chemicals to remove the original solvents and deodorize and bleach the oils. This process strips off most of the oils' nutritional value, including its defining properties, "sticky" and odor, followed by additional substances and vitamins to enrich it. Therefore, you can trust good traditional oils like mustard, groundnut, or gingelly (sesame) oil if ghee is not preferred. Many of the highest quality refined culinary oils are now pressed and refined without using chemical solvents, which is better than refined oil. Nevertheless, it is essential to remember that the calorific value of any oil is significantly higher than that of carbohydrates. Thus, moderation is vital, and there should be a daily limit on the amount of oil consumed unless coupled with a substantial amount of physical activity daily; excessive oil intake should be avoided.

Quantity of Food

Along with timely and quality eating, quantity is the third crucial parameter related to food. As the African proverb mentioned at the beginning of this chapter aptly puts it, in modern times, where physical activity is minimal, consuming one-fourth of our usual intake can be sufficient and healthy.

Determining the ideal quantity of daily intake is a relative matter. There is no one-size-fits-all approach, and fixed calorie limits like 1800 or 2400 calories a day are typically used for medical patients. An average person's decision should be based on their daily physical and mental activities. The goal is to feel energetic throughout the day without experiencing weakness or lethargy. If lethargy becomes a recurring issue, it might indicate an excessive intake of carbohydrates or sugars, resulting in a surplus of calories that are not being expended. This habit can lead to chronic illnesses and diseases, as seen in cases where people depend on sugary drinks to kickstart their work.

The quantity of food needed also depends on the type of work one engages in. For example, if you work in the field and require manual labor, your calorie intake will be higher. You will have more physical exertion because of your work, so your body will need to consume more food to keep the energy levels going. But if you do more mental work, you might need fewer calories. However, regardless of the nature of work, finding ways to expend the calories

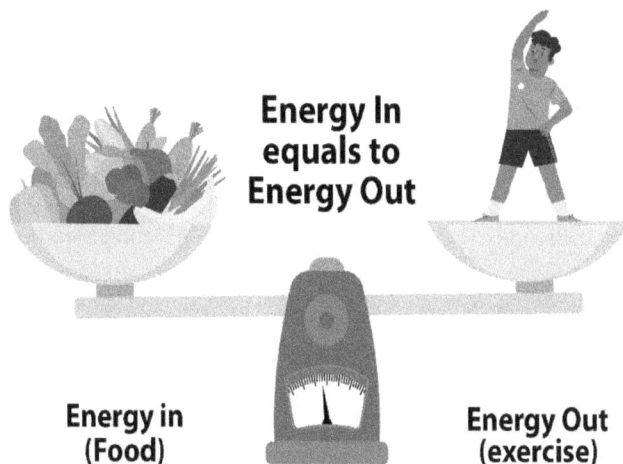

Energy In equals to Energy Out

Energy in (Food)

Energy Out (exercise)

> Importance of Food Consumption (eat) and food utilization (exercise) balance

consumed is essential, maintaining a balance between intake and expenditure. Moderation in food consumption is critical. Mindful eating practices can help individuals better understand their body's needs. Attention to hunger and satiety cues can prevent overeating and promote a healthier relationship with food. We must listen to our bodies and consume food when genuinely hungry rather than eating out of boredom, stress, or social pressure.

Incorporating nutrient-dense foods into our diets is vital for overall health. Fresh fruits, vegetables, whole grains, lean proteins, and healthy fats should form the foundation of our meals. These foods provide essential vitamins, minerals, and other micronutrients that support various bodily functions.

Optimal Fasting Practices

Fasting is an ancient practice with numerous health benefits. Different cultures have incorporated fasting in various forms, and modern trends, such as intermittent fasting, have gained popularity.

Fasting gives a much-needed break to the intestinal microbiota and triggers fat-burning after 14 to 18 hours of fasting. This process initially exhausts the stored glycogen in the liver, followed by lipolysis of excessive fats, which are stimuli for vascular inflammation in our body, aiding in weight loss. This provides the turnover of fat and glycogen. Additionally, fasting eliminates defective cells with the potential for malignant transformation by promoting apoptosis and preventing the growth of dangerous cancer cells.

The frequency of fasting depends on individual factors like body weight, work demands, and physical and mental needs. One fasting day per week is a good starting point, with more frequent fasting recommended for weight loss. Staying well-hydrated and avoiding calorie-containing products, including juices and sugary beverages, is vital during fasting.

Intermittent fasting has gained attention in recent years for its potential health benefits. This approach involves cycling between periods of eating and fasting. Popular methods include the 16/8 method, where one fasts for 16 hours and eats during an 8-hour window, and the 5:2 method, which involves eating normally for five days and restricting calorie intake to 500-600 calories on two non-consecutive days.

Studies have shown intermittent fasting may improve metabolic health, aid in weight loss, and extend lifespan. It can enhance insulin sensitivity, leading to better blood sugar control and reduced risk of type 2 diabetes. Additionally, fasting promotes *autophagy*, a natural cellular process that helps remove damaged cells and proteins, contributing to overall cellular health.

When adopting intermittent fasting, it is essential to do so under proper guidance and consider individual health conditions. Pregnant or breastfeeding women, individuals with a history of eating disorders, or those with certain medical conditions should approach fasting cautiously and consult healthcare professionals before starting any fasting regimen.

In conclusion, adjusting the timing, quality, and quantity of your food according to your lifestyle is essential for a healthy lifestyle. Attention to these three parameters can promote overall well-being and achieve a balanced and nourishing diet. Moderation, mindful eating, and incorporating nutrient-dense foods are vital to fostering good eating habits. Furthermore, incorporating intermittent fasting under proper guidance can provide potential health benefits and contribute to a healthier and happier life. Remember, it is essential to prioritize your well-being, and a thoughtful approach to food can significantly impact your overall health and longevity.

Nutraceutical Myths and Misconceptions

Regarding overall healthy foods and diets, it's crucial to recognize the influence of genetics and geographical location. Observational studies often focus on individuals consuming specific diets in particular regions, but we must be cautious not to accept their results as absolute truth unquestioningly. Most of the studies are observational, and conducting Randomized control trials with nutraceutical product always have confounder and compliance issues. Moreover, many of these studies may have vested interests, promoting them for their own direct or indirect benefit.

A prime example of a misleading concept is the belief that fish oil reduces vessel inflammation and heart diseases. This conclusion was drawn from the longevity of a specific population in Greenland: the Eskimos, who consume fish and omega-3 fatty acid, which is associated with longevity. However, attributing their health solely to fish oil ignores other crucial factors, such as their overall lifestyle, diet, and environmental influences. This association has yet to be replicated in other populations, raising doubts about the validity of this claim. Promoting fish oil as a solution for heart disease is anecdotal and highly questionable. No doubt fish in diet has a beneficial effect, but fish oil has equivalent benefit as taking fish is incorrect.

Nutraceuticals are another area where unreliable concepts and products prevail. Marketed as new-age pharmaceutical capsules acting as dietary supplements, they need proper regulation and proof of their proclaimed heart health or overall health benefits. These products should be approached with caution as their effectiveness remains uncertain.

Lastly, it is essential to recognize that there is no one-size-fits-all approach to nutrition. No specific food or diet can be universally deemed beneficial for all individuals. Instead, our health is influenced by our good habits and the consistency with which we practice them. Emphasizing healthy and consistent dietary choices is paramount for overall well-being.

Food, Energy & Heart Health

When we consume food, our bodies break down the macronutrients of carbohydrates and fats. Carbohydrates are broken into glucose, while fats are broken into fatty acids. Both glucose and fatty acids undergo the oxidation process, combining with oxygen to generate energy from Adenosine Triphosphates (ATPs). ATPs serve as the energy currency within living beings, powering various cellular metabolisms.

Fatty acids have an advantage over glucose in ATP production, yielding more ATPs per unit. Different organs use glucose and fatty acids in varying proportions. For instance, the brain heavily relies on glucose to produce energy, while the heart predominantly utilizes fatty acids, using only a tiny percentage of glucose and sometimes proteins when necessary. Therefore, the heart doesn't primarily depend on carbohydrates for its functioning. However, if the brain does not receive a supply of glucose through the bloodstream, it can lead to unconsciousness.

On the other hand, the heart can switch between glucose and fatty acids depending on the body's needs. This adaptability occurs when there is a deficiency of fats or an excess of glucose, such as in cases of diabetes. These metabolic changes can reduce the heart's efficiency and cause abnormalities. For individuals with diabetes, these changes pose the first risk to the heart. The second problem arises from decreased oxygen levels, which can also occur due to diabetes. As mentioned earlier, glucose and fatty acids require oxygen to produce ATPs. The heart, a primary organ that works continuously, requires substantial oxygen to generate ATPs for pumping. Reduced oxygen levels can lead to decreased energy production in the heart, resulting in weakened pumping and potential heart diseases over time.

It is essential to be mindful of our diet to maintain heart health. While no specific foods or diets are categorized as solely good for heart health, an excessive intake of fats can be detrimental. Excessive fatty acids can be deposited at various locations in the heart, causing inflammation and increasing stickiness of the endothelium, the inner lining of blood vessels, and heart chambers. The vascular inflammation set in by fat deposits impairs the endothelial cell's neutral behavior to become sticky, attracting leukocyte cells, part of our immune system in the blood. This sticky endothelium creates a portal for fats to enter and form foam cells, which are the initial stages of atherosclerosis. These foam cells can emerge from the sub-endothelium and obstruct blood circulation, leading to cardiovascular diseases.

Atherosclerosis can affect various arteries supplying the brain, heart, intestines, and lower limbs. However, the brain and heart, highly functional organs, are more susceptible to atherosclerosis due to their higher blood flow and oxygen demand.

Maintaining a balanced diet and lifestyle is crucial, avoiding excessive consumption of fats and promoting regular physical activity to promote heart health. Additionally, managing diabetes and ensuring adequate oxygen supply to the heart is essential for reducing the risk of heart diseases and maintaining overall cardiovascular well-being. By making conscious choices about our diet and lifestyle, we can protect our hearts and lead healthier lives.

Food Myths and Misconceptions

This is an era where we are overloaded with information from various sources. The allure of quick-fix diets and trendy health fads is undeniable. The vast expanse of the internet inundates us with an avalanche of dietary advice. Based on the information available on the internet, many individuals impulsively switch their eating habits without fully comprehending the potential consequences. A prime example is the sudden surge in people adopting olive oil as their go-to cooking oil after reading about its purported health benefits online. However, they need to grasp that using olive oil correctly is essential for reaping its advantages, and misusing it can lead to unexpected health problems.

Another prevalent trend is the high-protein, low-carb ketogenic diet, which has gained immense popularity for aiding weight loss. Many people, lured by the promise of quick results, dive headlong into this restrictive diet, eliminating carbohydrates and overindulging in proteins and fats. In the initial weeks, they may revel in their apparent weight loss success, but a closer look at their lipid profiles might reveal alarming levels of cholesterol and triglycerides. Additionally, they might feel pervasive fatigue and listlessness as their body struggles to adjust to this abrupt dietary shift. The truth is that this diet, like many others propagated on social media, may only be suitable for some, especially considering that we have been conditioned to eat a particular way since childhood.

The human body is a complex, finely tuned machine, and dramatic changes to its nutritional intake can throw it off balance, impacting both physical and mental health. These diets can inadvertently promote a sedentary lifestyle, as the body struggles to cope with the lack of essential nutrients and energy. When we encounter patients who have undergone such misguided diet changes, we emphasize the importance of making gradual, sustainable adjustments to their eating habits. Instead of adopting restrictive diets, we advocate for a balanced approach to food, focusing on the timing, quality, and quantity of the meals.

Investing in good habits becomes the cornerstone of achieving lasting health and well-being. We refer to this investment as a dedication to health, a conscious effort to nurture our bodies and minds through mindful eating. Choosing quality foods, consuming in a time-restricted manner to allow for proper digestion, and avoiding late-night eating are fundamental aspects of this dedication. Balancing our food intake with our daily physical and mental demands ensures that we feel energized and vibrant throughout the day.

In contrast to the belief that good health can be achieved up to a certain age and then forgotten, we must realize that the modern world presents new challenges that necessitate consistent efforts to maintain good health. Pesticides in our food and environmental pollution have made us more susceptible to diseases, necessitating a proactive approach to our well-being. By embracing healthy eating habits and regular exercise, we fortify our bodies to withstand the onslaught of potential health risks.

In conclusion, pursuing optimal health is not a fleeting endeavor but a lifelong journey. Discernment and mindfulness should be our guiding principles when navigating the vast landscape of online dietary advice. Instead of chasing after quick-fix diets, we should invest in building sustainable and nourishing habits. By understanding the impact of our nutritional choices on our bodies and minds, we empower ourselves to lead joyful, fulfilling lives. Our health is a treasure that requires dedicated attention, and by making informed decisions about what we consume, we can unlock the potential for a vibrant and thriving existence.❖

5

EXERCISE & HEALTH INVESTMENT

"Exercise makes time not takes time."

- A Popular Saying

Many individuals begin exercising from a young age, influenced by their parents, relatives, or friends. This early exposure to discipline makes it easier for them to embrace physical, mental, and spiritual exercises later in life. However, others may only see the necessity of training once they reach a certain age, making it more challenging to find the motivation to start.

Many people get the motivation to exercise after they have developed a disease. The fear of worsening their condition or facing a relapse can drive them to exercise for a while, but they may eventually become lethargic. Such individuals require a significant mental push, starting with small tasks and gradually building on them.

Exercise encompasses more than just physical activity, and it is crucial to comprehend the three essential dimensions of exercise for optimizing our well-being and embracing the gift of life to its fullest. Physical, mental, and spiritual practices form an interwoven tapestry that, when harmoniously integrated, nurtures a healthy heart, a robust body, and a joy-filled existence.

Physical Exercises

Physical exercise encompasses various activities, from purposeful exercises such as walking, jogging, running, dancing, or swimming to daily household chores. Engaging in any bodily movement expends energy, burning ATPs or calories while promoting increased blood flow. There are two primary categories of exercises based on how you exercise and the energy expended.

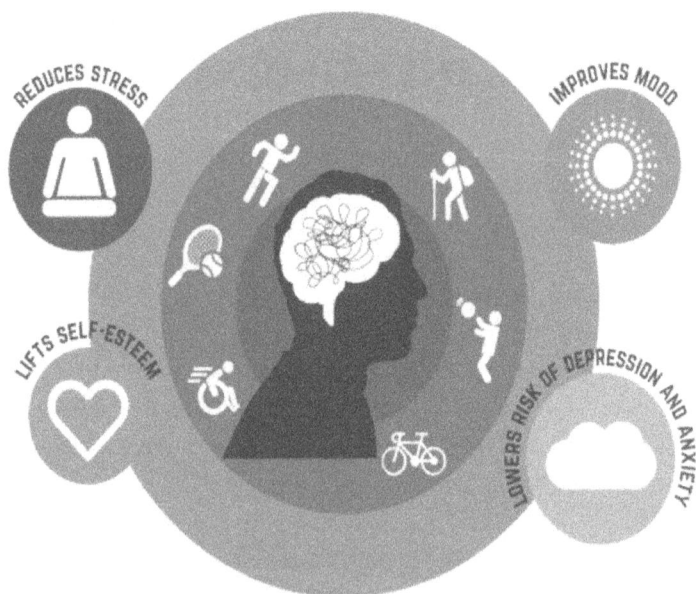

Impact of Physical Activity on Mental Health

The first category is isometric exercises, which involve maintaining specific positions to strengthen and stabilize muscles without joint movement or bending. On the other hand, isotonic exercises include movements like squats, pushups, bench presses, and deadlifts, as well as aerobic exercises like walking, running, hiking, dancing, and swimming. Isotonic exercises help maintain strength and aid muscle building, making them essential to any workout routine. Additionally, there are isokinetic exercises that involve using specialized machines to exercise. However, in practical terms, they are similar to isotonic exercises, exerting more pressure on muscles to facilitate muscle growth and development.

The Connection Between Heart Disease and Exercise

Selecting a suitable exercise class is essential for a person's physical needs, work constraints, and potential limitations due to injuries or illnesses. Generally, aerobic exercises are considered beneficial for most individuals, as they contribute to overall well-being and health. An excellent physical exercise routine is highly recommended unless a specific medical condition is diagnosed.

Regarding heart-related diseases, four specific conditions require a doctor's evaluation before engaging in any exercise routine. These conditions are Hypertrophic Cardiomyopathy (HCM), Arrhythmogenic Right Ventricular Dysplasia (ARVD), Catecholaminergic Polymorphic Ventricular Tachycardia (CPVT), and certain Channelopathies, such as Long QT syndrome (LQTS). LQTS is an arrhythmic condition where the heart appears normal, but the patient may experience life-threatening rhythm disorders leading to cardiac arrest and even death. An ECG and ECHO cardiogram are the minimum to be done in the suspected case of the above diseases. Individuals with these conditions and those with a family history of such diseases should undergo early medical evaluations and take preventive measures, as these conditions often have genetic links. A careful assessment of symptoms and family medical history can help rule out these conditions.

Exercise and impact on the coronary block

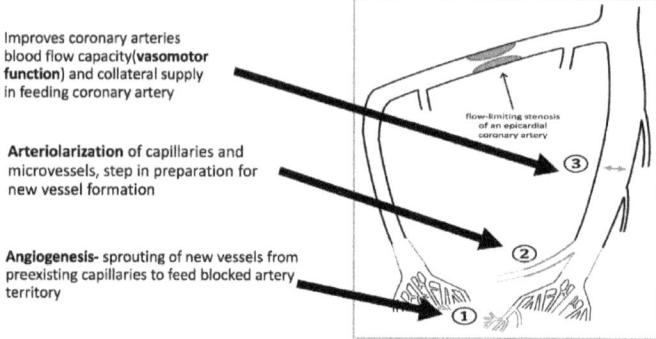

Improves coronary arteries blood flow capacity(**vasomotor function**) and collateral supply in feeding coronary artery

Arteriolarization of capillaries and microvessels, step in preparation for new vessel formation

Angiogenesis- sprouting of new vessels from preexisting capillaries to feed blocked artery territory

flow-limiting stenosis of an epicardial coronary artery

Apart from the mentioned four diseases, other heart patients, including those with a history of heart failure, Coronary Artery Disease (CAD), or previous stenting, are recommended to participate in exercises under the supervision of a doctor, particularly in the initial stages. Medical professionals or cardiac rehabilitation personnel can monitor heart function, lung capacity, and other essential systems during exercise to determine the appropriate activity level. Regular physical exercise is advised for heart patients, in addition to their medications, as it aids in maintaining heart health and minimizing the risk of disease recurrence or associated factors.

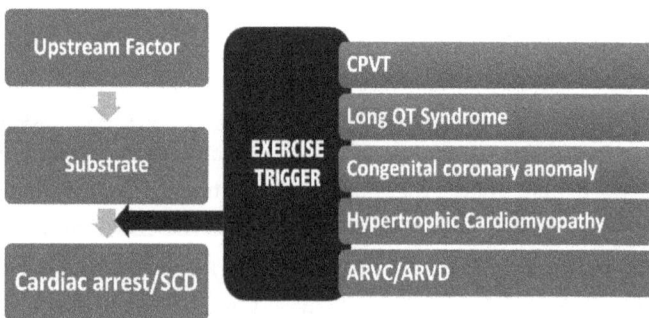

Upstream Factor → Substrate → Cardiac arrest/SCD

EXERCISE TRIGGER

- CPVT
- Long QT Syndrome
- Congenital coronary anomaly
- Hypertrophic Cardiomyopathy
- ARVC/ARVD

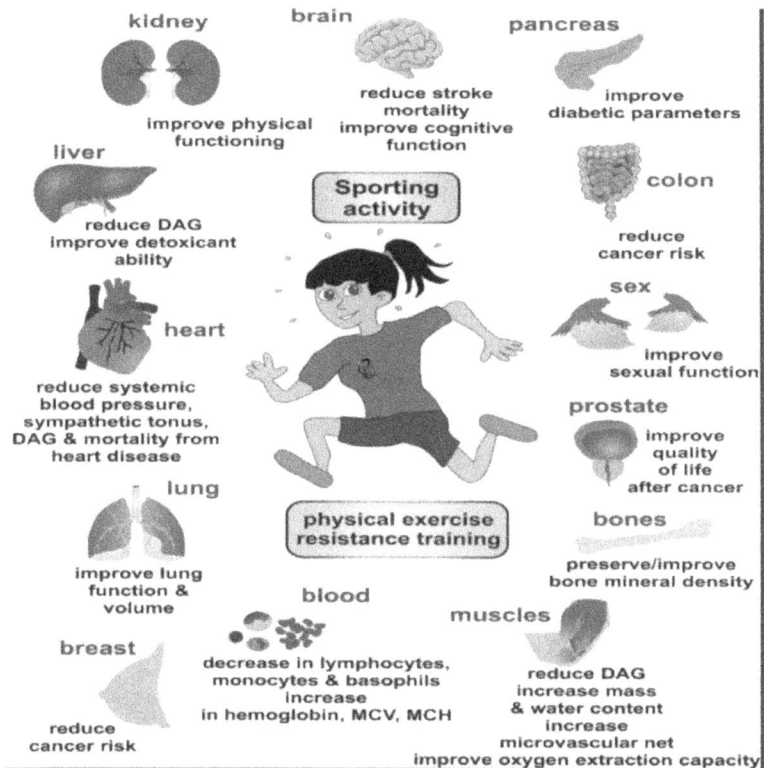

kidney — improve physical functioning

brain — reduce stroke mortality improve cognitive function

pancreas — improve diabetic parameters

liver — reduce DAG improve detoxicant ability

Sporting activity

colon — reduce cancer risk

sex — improve sexual function

heart — reduce systemic blood pressure, sympathetic tonus, DAG & mortality from heart disease

prostate — improve quality of life after cancer

lung — improve lung function & volume

physical exercise resistance training

bones — preserve/improve bone mineral density

blood — decrease in lymphocytes, monocytes & basophils increase in hemoglobin, MCV, MCH

muscles — reduce DAG increase mass & water content increase microvascular net improve oxygen extraction capacity

breast — reduce cancer risk

Exercise is Hormone for Health

Physical exercise plays a crucial role in the lives of both healthy individuals and those with medical conditions. If you aspire to enjoy a healthy life, incorporating exercise is vital, and you can choose the type of exercise that resonates with you. Whether it's dancing, swimming, playing badminton, lawn tennis, or any other activity you are passionate about, engaging in it regularly can be an enjoyable way to stay fit. Physical exercises and timely, quality food are the best preventive medicine against heart-related diseases, contributing to a healthier and happier life.

Mental Exercise

Throughout history, numerous leaders have emerged in various fields who excelled in their skills and lived longer, lasting lasting impact on society. One common characteristic that sets them apart is their insatiable thirst for learning and willingness to take on challenges. These leaders were never content with mediocrity; instead, they consistently pushed themselves to perform to the best of their abilities and contributed selflessly to society. As a result, their learnings and contributions to the community yielded tremendous returns later in their lives. The annals of history are filled with such exemplary leaders, and a recent example is Dr. APJ Abdul Kalam, who continued to work passionately until the remarkable age of 92. From his early days in the DRDO to becoming one of India's top scientists and eventually serving as the President of the country, Dr. Kalam's dedication to learning and growth was awe-inspiring. Despite heart-related challenges, he remained an avid learner and consistently challenged himself.

The habit of actively learning new things and embracing challenges is a secret mental exercise that elevates a person's capabilities. It is a vital need for every individual to keep their mind engaged and growing. Such mental exercises also lay the foundation for practical physical work, creating a healthy and balanced environment. The combined activeness of mind and body indirectly benefits blood circulation and all other systems within the body. Whether the learning or challenge is significant or minor, it builds strong willpower and a resilient spirit. You may have noticed that many government employees are surrounded by several diseases just a few years after retirement from a government job, particularly those who stop working in their role. The most common reason is physical inactivity and lack of mild to moderate mental challenges at workplaces, which keep them from developing modern epidemic diseases like diabetes and other chronic diseases.

Learning is a mental exercise that demands focus, patience, and perseverance. When surrounded by negativity, actively learning something new can counterbalance the effects of pessimism, infusing positivity into one's life. Besides physical exercises, dedicating time to learning and embracing new challenges helps keep the mind sharp, body systems active, and spirits youthful.

Embracing the habit of constant learning and willingly confronting challenges is a powerful mental exercise that enhances a person's overall well-being. It is a building block for personal growth, resilience, and an optimistic outlook, all contributing to a healthier and more fulfilling life. As we navigate life's journey, let us remember that the thirst for knowledge and the eagerness to face new challenges are invaluable tools to nurture a vibrant mind and body.

Spiritual Exercise

Spirituality is an exercise that revolves around understanding yourself, your place, and your purpose in the vast universe. After physical and mental exercises, spiritual exercise takes you to a higher level, building your inner mental strength. Contrary to common misconceptions, spirituality is not confined to following a religion, God, or godman. Spirituality is a stable foundation against uncertainties and low points in life, guiding you through life's journey and empowering you with strength and focus. It becomes a steady base upon which you can perform your physical and mental activities more effectively.

To embark on a spiritual journey, you need not look further than what you are doing now – questioning. You initiate your spiritual quest by questioning things and yourself, such as the purpose of your existence, your unique talents, and the path to genuine happiness. While religious books and individuals who have trodden the spiritual path can offer guidance, it is essential to forge your perspective, allowing room for self-correction. As you delve deeply into contemplation, you will begin to comprehend the society and embrace broader concepts like 'Vasudaiva Kutumbam,' the Indian cultural philosophy that proclaims all people in the world belong to one family.

You may wonder how spirituality relates to your health, but once again, it is an exercise that grants you mental peace. Streamlining your thoughts spiritually harmonizes your interactions with people and the world at the micro or macro level. You become attuned to nature and find harmony in your relationships and surroundings. As a result, navigating through difficult situations becomes smoother and less turbulent.

Spirituality offers ample mental training, helping you discern meaning in every aspect of life. When faced with physical or mental challenges, your spiritual stamina becomes your core strength, guiding you through adversities and preserving your resilience.

युक्ताहारविहारस्य युक्तचेष्टस्य कर्मसु ।
युक्तस्वप्नावबोधस्य योगो भवति दुःखहा ।। 17।।

yuktāhāra-vihārasya yukta-cheṣṭasya karmasu
yukta-svapnāvabodhasya yogo bhavati duḥkha-hā

Bhagavad Gita 6.17: But those who are temperate in eating and recreation, balanced in work, and regulated in sleep, can mitigate all sorrows by practicing Yog.

Engaging in physical, mental, and spiritual exercises will empower you to build strength and a robust personality. When confronting formidable challenges, the combined force of these exercises illuminates the path ahead. All three practices are crucial throughout life, and their strength is intertwined with the heart, as emphasized in the earlier chapter, highlighting the profound connection between the brain and the heart. The activities occurring in your brain indirectly impact the vitality of your heart and body, reinforcing the importance of nurturing all aspects of your being for a fulfilling and healthy life.

Health Insurance Vs Health Investment

As a developing country, India has made progress in recognizing the importance of health insurance, providing coverage for individuals when they fall ill. However, a more progressive approach would focus on preventive measures to minimize illness and promote a healthier society. This can be achieved through incentives or policies encouraging healthy habits and lifestyles.

The premium paid to insurance companies to cover them for the disease in the future is called health premium, and all developed countries have adopted it. In European countries, it is surrounded by government. It has created a new face of the health sector as a new business, which is a deciding factor in the cost of treatment in hospitals empaneled by insurance companies. In India, health insurance coverage is minimal but growing by government and private companies.

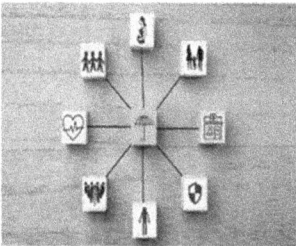

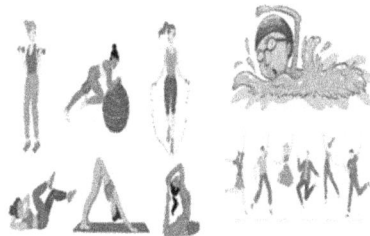

> **Difference in Health Insurance and Health Investment (we need both)**

"Health Investment" is a word I am currently coining in this book for the first time for all the habits and measures to prevent diseases in our capacity. I have coined this for the purpose.

It is an individual's *investment* for being healthy. It is *time* for health, which includes exercise, lifestyle modification, and prevention of burnout in the present scenario. It is a daily investment in these habits. It is *not a capital investment*. It is a time investment in the practices that prevent diseases. Jogging for 45 minutes daily, 300 days a year, is a health investment. There are many ways to invest in health investment. We have to find how we want to invest. The most important myth is that we do not have time for exercise. But a simple fact to remember is that exercise doesn't consume your time but *makes time*. When you teach exercise in your daily routine, the time you invest in exercise helps increase your physical and mental efficiency. It reduces the time you usually take to complete the work and saves time.

Countries like Japan have implemented administration-level checks on employee lifestyles, where unhealthy habits can lead to reduced perks and disapproval of promotions. Such measures create awareness and incentivize people to stay fit and healthy. In contrast, in countries without such norms, like India, we see a rising prevalence of obesity, hypertension, and diabetes. While genetic or accident-related reasons may warrant some leeway, encouraging a healthy lifestyle will provide valuable data on the impact of genetics on specific populations, aiding healthcare understanding and planning.

Incentivizing employees to spend time with their families and friends and incorporating this into the working culture would significantly improve community health. When people are rewarded for their well-being, others will be motivated to strive for the same, resulting in a win-win situation.

Another vital aspect of fostering a healthier society is encouraging physical activity and regular exercise. Creating accessible and safe spaces for outdoor activities, promoting sports at schools, and organizing community fitness events can inspire people to engage in regular physical exercise. Workplace wellness programs can also play a significant role in motivating employees to adopt active lifestyles. By incorporating exercise breaks or offering fitness incentives, companies can contribute to the overall well-being of their workforce.

Nutrition is also pivotal in maintaining heart health and preventing cardiovascular diseases. Encouraging a balanced diet rich in fruits, vegetables, whole grains, and lean proteins while limiting the intake of processed foods and excessive sugars can positively impact heart health. Educational campaigns on healthy eating habits can help individuals make informed choices.

Furthermore, mental health is interconnected with physical health; stress management is essential for overall well-being. Encouraging stress-relief techniques such as meditation, mindfulness, or yoga can help individuals cope with the pressures of modern life. Prioritizing mental health in workplace environments and providing access to mental health resources can significantly improve employee morale and productivity.

One of the most crucial policy interventions needed is addressing the late-night working culture prevalent in the Indian workforce catering to European and US establishments or clients. Continuous late-night work deprives individuals of proper rest, leading to increased stress and a toxic environment. Collaborating with industry giants, the government should implement norms to minimize or avoid late-night work as much as possible. It is essential to create a working culture that prioritizes employee well-being and includes breaks for rejuvenation.

In recent times, India has taken steps toward health insurance. But that alone is not good enough because further emphasis on preventive measures, incentivizing healthy habits, promoting genetic awareness, and addressing late-night working practices play a vital role in building a healthier society. By actively pursuing such policy decisions and fostering a culture of health-consciousness, we can safeguard the well-being of our youth and promote a healthier future for all. A multi-faceted approach that combines physical, mental, and genetic health interventions will pave the way for a thriving and resilient society where individuals can lead fulfilling lives free from the burden of preventable illnesses.

DR. ASHUTOSH KUMAR

SECTION-B

6

HEART DISEASE CLASSIFICATIONS & NORMS

"I think... if it is true that there are as many minds as there are heads, then there are as many kinds of love as there are hearts."

— Leo Tolstoy

In the preceding section of this book, we have extensively explored the various factors that influence both heart health and overall well-being. In this section, we will thoroughly examine heart diseases, encompassing their classifications, different treatment procedures,

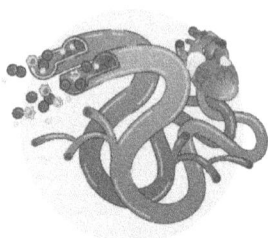

Cardiovascular disease

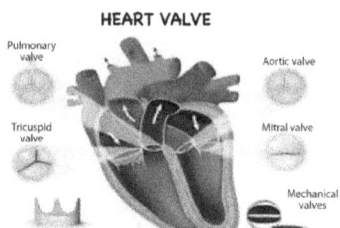

Valvular disease

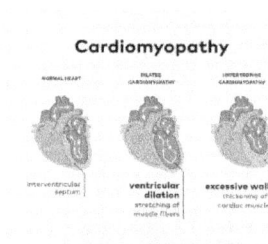

Muscle disease

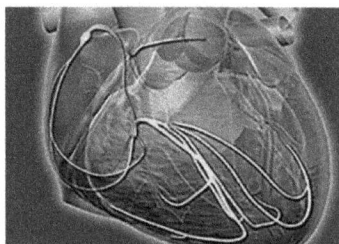

Electric disease-arrhythmia

Types of Heart Disease

and universally embraced norms.

Classes of Heart Diseases: Heart diseases can be classified into **four main classes**. The first class comprises coronary artery diseases **(CAD)**, which are related to the Coronary arteries responsible for supplying blood to the heart. The second class includes Valvular Heart Diseases **(VHD)**, which affect the heart valves. The third class encompasses **Myocardial or Muscle Diseases (cardiomyopathies)** associated with the heart muscles. Finally, the fourth class contains **Electrical diseases or Arrhythmias**, characterized by problems with the heart's electrical system. These four classifications provide a comprehensive overview of heart-related disorders.

Moreover, as we have studied earlier, the heart is an efficient motor. Still, to function most efficiently, the various functions (vascular, valvular, muscle, and electrical activity) are orchestrated in a very coordinated manner. They all are hinged here and there to provide the most efficient pump function 24/7, 365 days a year throughout life. Any stress or derangement in one function will certainly affect another function and ultimately taxes the cardiac efficiency if not corrected in a time-sensitive manner by lifestyle modifications, drugs, and sometimes interventions (surgical or nonsurgical). It means that a disease from one class at its outset can enter another type of heart disease over time. This creates a possibility of permutations and combinations of these diseases in heart patients. For instance, a patient may initially experience Coronary Artery Disease, followed by the development of muscle disease, which we call cardiomyopathy. Since it happens in patients already diagnosed with CAD, we call it ischemic cardiomyopathy. Later, the same patient can have ventricular tachycardia due to the scar formation during the initial heart attack. Hence, the same patient has entered the fourth class of disease called arrhythmia. Over time, this patient initially developed a heart attack(myocardial infarction), leading to muscle weakness(myocardial dysfunction) due to late presentation.

Finally, the scar formed due to fibrosis of the dead myocardium during the initial heart attack, which lead to scar-related ventricular tachycardia. The timeline of disease in a person is very individual. It has many factors, including genetics. That's why it becomes essential to understand that trial-based information should not be imposed on an index case when making a conclusion or prognosis. Every patient is different and unique in the course and timeline of their disease. Due to this complexity, each case requires an accurate diagnosis to identify the primary or initiating illness. Pinpointing the specific components, such as valves, muscles, electrical systems, or coronaries, that are affected initially is crucial for understanding disease progression.

Heart patients may present with diverse symptoms over time due to the coexistence of multiple diseases in various permutations and combinations. For instance, a patient may initially experience breathlessness, which later evolves into giddiness when the electrical system becomes affected. A patient's medical history guides diagnosis and treatment decisions in this context. It helps medical professionals determine the initial disease and comprehend how other issues have developed and contributed to its progression. With this knowledge, physicians can tailor each patient to appropriate and personalized treatment plans, optimizing their chances of a successful outcome.

Course of Heart Disease

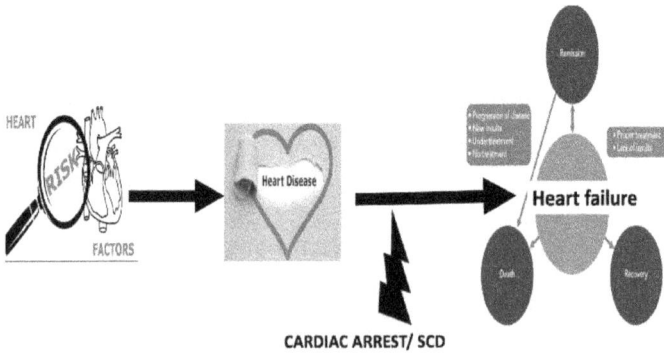

The Course of Heart Disease

Any Heart disease can progress to a condition called Heart failure. It means that the heart cannot pump blood around the body properly. It usually happens because the heart has become too weak or stiff. It is the final destination of all heart disease, from vascular to valvular. In the story of some heart diseases with particular risk factors, these are episodes of cardiac emergency called heart attack or cardiac arrest. They should be treated urgently to save the life of the patient.

Heart Failure

Indeed, all heart abnormalities, maladaptation for a prolonged time, or disease that impairs cardiac function in any way compounded over time **impairs** heart pumping efficiency, which, in medical terminology, we label as *heart failure*. However, it is essential to understand that heart failure does not imply that the heart has entirely ceased to function. Instead, it refers to a state where the heart pumping function is impaired and unable to function at maximum efficiency. Consequently, the heart cannot pump enough blood to maintain the body's overall metabolism and function properly.

In heart failure, the heart cannot meet the body's demands for oxygen and nutrients, leading to various symptoms and complications. The reduced pumping capacity can result from a wide range of heart diseases, including issues related to the heart valves (valvular), heart muscles (myocardial), coronary arteries (coronary), and electrical system (arrhythmias).

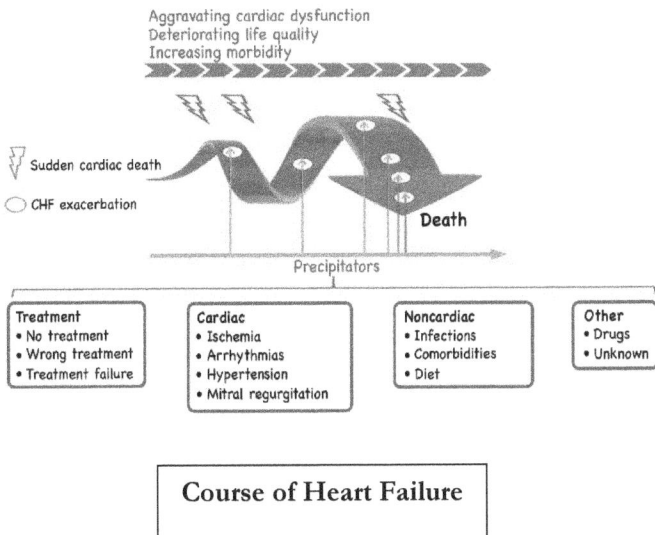

Aggravating cardiac dysfunction
Deteriorating life quality
Increasing morbidity

Sudden cardiac death

CHF exacerbation

Death

Precipitators

Treatment	Cardiac	Noncardiac	Other
• No treatment	• Ischemia	• Infections	• Drugs
• Wrong treatment	• Arrhythmias	• Comorbidities	• Unknown
• Treatment failure	• Hypertension	• Diet	
	• Mitral regurgitation		

Course of Heart Failure

When the heart has trouble with its electrical signals or pumping blood, it cannot correctly move blood all around the body. This means that organs and tissues might not get enough oxygen and nutrients, making a person feel tired and out of breath. These problems are part of what's called heart failure.

It is essential to understand that heart failure is a serious issue that needs to be taken seriously. People can feel better and prevent more problems with the proper medical care and treatments. Getting diagnosed early, making lifestyle changes, and following the doctor's advice are essential to manage heart failure and its causes. By caring for heart problems and ensuring the heart works well, people can have a better chance of living a healthy and good life.

Two killer Cardiac Emergencies (Heart Attack & Cardiac Arrest)

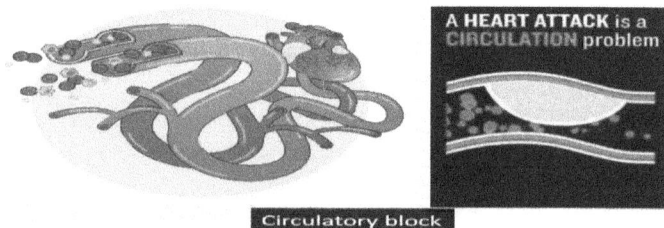

Circulatory block

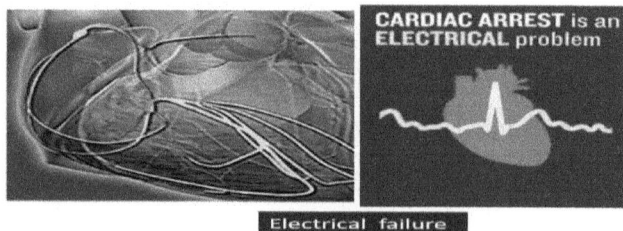

Electrical failure

Difference in Heart Attack and Cardiac Arrest

Two cardiac emergencies are often confused by the patient's need for differentiation. One is due to vascular compromise, while the other is an electrical abnormality. This emergency can lead to sudden deterioration of the cardiac pump, leading to heart failure to a cardiac standstill, and is lethal if not attended urgently. If the cardiac pump function is impaired due to the obstruction in the cardiac circulation of blood (coronary artery block), it is called Heart Attack, medically known as *Myocardial Infarction (MI)*. During a Heart Attack, a part of the heart muscle is deprived of sufficient blood supply, a condition called Ischemia. The affected portion of the heart muscle may eventually die due to compromised blood circulation, a condition called infarction.

During a Heart Attack, the heart's blood circulation is severely reduced or blocked, causing pain and discomfort. The duration and severity of symptoms can vary. Most of the time, patients are very symptomatic. Still, in some patients, it may be minor chest discomfort, which may go unnoticed or overlooked because the block is in a minor branch not supplying a large territory of the heart, unlike the major branch coronary artery block. Sometimes, it depends on the patient's bearing capacity. In about 25-50% of patients, *auto thrombolysis* (clot dissolution without drug/intervention) can spontaneously relieve the patient's pain. During this time, when a coronary artery is blocked, the territory it supplies will lose function in addition to chest pain. Still, the remaining territory of the other coronary will be taking care of the heart pumping function. Hence, the heart is still beating and trying to pump blood, albeit with weakened power.

On the other hand, Cardiac Arrest is an electrical phenomenon where cardiac pump function is deranged due to electrical underpinning. Suppose the heartbeat goes very fast, particularly in the lower chamber, as it happens in ventricular tachycardia or ventricular fibrillation. In that case, it leads to a cardiac standstill, also called *asystole*, a life-threatening condition. This type of cardiac arrest is also called Tachy Cardiac arrest. Similarly, heart beating, if it goes very slow, will again compromise cardiac pump function, and we use the word Bradycardiac arrest, which occurs when the heart stops receiving electrical impulses necessary for its functioning. Understanding that a heart attack can progress to cardiac arrest if the blood flow remains obstructed is crucial. It usually happens in the initial hours of a heart attack. Statistics show that around 25% of patients who experience a heart attack and cannot reach the hospital die of cardiac arrest. The lack of blood supply during a heart attack can cause electrical abnormalities in the heart, leading to cardiac arrest.

Cardiac arrest is a transient phase between life and death, where the heart stops functioning. However, it is called a transient phase because the heart can still be resuscitated after cardiac arrest through medical interventions such as CPR (Cardiopulmonary Resuscitation) and electric shocks. CPR involves chest compressions to maintain circulation and oxygenation till the heart regains its autonomous beating activity. The timely administration of CPR and electric shocks can potentially restart the heart and save a person's life.

In summary, a Heart Attack results from blocked coronary circulation, a vascular phenomenon, while Cardiac Arrest is due to an acute and severe electrical system dysfunction. Both conditions are life-endangering and require immediate medical attention and intervention to increase the chances of survival and minimize potential complications.

Deadly Duo-Cardiac Arrest in Heart Attack

When someone has a heart attack, their heart can go through many other complications, affecting the heart's rhythm adversely or impacting the way its valves work. The first hours after a heart attack are the most risky for having serious rhythm problems. These problems can include dangerous heart rhythms like ventricular tachycardia and ventricular fibrillation, which can be harmful and even deadly. These are the main reasons some people die suddenly after a heart attack, either at home or on the way to the hospital.

In some cases, the heart's normal electrical signals can have issues. This can cause problems with how the upper and lower heart chambers communicate. This is like a problem with the heart's electrical system, particularly the AV node(heart transmitter). The lower chambers(ventricle), which are responsible for ejecting the blood to the whole body, may not receive the current generated in the upper chamber, and the heart's beating can slow down, causing symptoms like dizziness, fainting, and in the worst case, even stopping altogether. To fix this, doctors might need to use a temporary pacemaker (TPI) device to help the heart beat normally.

I once treated a 45-year-old guy who works in the IT industry. He was just casually playing badminton when suddenly, he started sweating like he was in a sauna. His chest felt tight, and he knew something was not right. So, he takes a breather, sits down, and hopes the discomfort disappears. But it doesn't. Now, he is an occasional smoker; to top it off, his family has a history of heart troubles. It's like the heart disease lottery; his family drew the short straw on the paternal side.

Things started to take a terrifying turn when he was rushed to the hospital in an ambulance. The ECG machine is plugged in, monitoring his heart's every beat. And then, out of the blue, he's drenched in sweat again, and the world starts spinning. Next thing you know, he's out cold. Thank goodness for that ECG machine because it spotted a nasty villain called Ventricular Tachycardia (VT) making a mess of his heart rhythm, and it's a one-way ticket to chaos called Ventricular Fibrillation. The medical team took prompt action, giving him a DC shock, and he sprang back to life. But this isn't the end; he has three more rounds with VT, and the shock is his lifeline each time. Finally, once they got him to the hospital, we rushed him to the Cathlab. A closer look reveals that his Left Anterior Descending artery is playing hide-and-seek behind a big, bad clot. We immediately performed an angioplasty and put in a stent to save his heart from further damage.

Fast forward, and he's on the road to recovery and released from the hospital in 3 days, returning to his IT job. Here's the lesson: without that ambulance equipped with a cardioversion setup, he might not have made it to the hospital in one piece. It's a reminder that sometimes, technology and quick action are the real superheroes.

Narrow window of Opportunity & Cardiac Arrest

When a person's heart function stops, they die. When the heart stops beating or contracting, blood circulation is severely impacted. Without blood flow, none of the organs can survive for long. In the case of other organs, there may be a chance for survival. For example, if the lungs stop functioning, a patient can be put on a ventilator to assist with breathing.

Similarly, if the brain experiences an interruption in function, the patient may still survive without immediate mental capabilities, and recovery could be possible. However, if the heart fails to pump blood, all the organs will soon cease functioning. The brain is the first to be affected, unconscious within 10 to 30 seconds after blood circulation interruption. This leads to the patient fainting and collapsing. Soon after, the respiratory system also becomes compromised, resulting in a combined cardiac and respiratory arrest, known as cardiopulmonary arrest. The heart's electrical activity must be restored as quickly as possible to keep a person alive in this critical situation.

During a cardiac arrest, the index case or person is hanging between life and death with a narrow window of opportunity to revive them to life by CPR if done as early as possible. A cardiac arrest can have two possible courses. In some cases, acute life-threatening killer rhythm terminates spontaneously, aborting cardiac arrest followed by spontaneous recovery of the person to life. This scenario is called "spontaneously recovered cardiac arrest," where the patient experiences a cardiac arrest and eventually recovers without any external assistance. However, in most reported cases, a patient experiencing cardiac arrest will receive immediate cardiopulmonary resuscitation (CPR) and, if necessary, electric shocks. This resuscitation process can continue for several minutes until the patient regains breathing and the heart regains its beating. In such instances, it is termed "resuscitated cardiac arrest." CPR involves chest compressions to help the heart pump blood to all the organs when it's not working correctly. Sometimes, it works and brings the person back, but other times it might not. If CPR is started quickly, there's a better chance of revival to life. If the person begins breathing and their heartbeat returns, they might recover independently or with medical help. But if their breathing and heartbeat don't return, they might not survive. So, a person can either get better on their own, with help, or unfortunately not make it.

CPR (Cardiopulmonary Resuscitation)

When someone suddenly passes out, the first thing to do is check if they're breathing. If they're not living and you can't feel their heartbeat or pulse, they're having a cardiac arrest, which is dire. To help in this emergency, you need to do cardiopulmonary resuscitation or CPR. The main focus of CPR is pressing on the chest firmly and at a certain pace. The old way of giving breaths into their mouth is not commonly used. The idea is to press on the chest hard and fast to push blood around the body and to the brain. This helps the heart start working again. It might need to be strong enough to break a rib or two, but that's okay because it's important to get the heart pumping again. Doing CPR this way can help restore the heart's normal function in about half to three-quarters of cases when it's done quickly. CPR also gives time for the person to get to the hospital.

I once treated a 65-year-old man who collapsed dramatically in his house. He was in a heated argument with his wife, and things were getting loud. Suddenly, he collapses, and he's out cold with no breathing. He was incredibly lucky as his son is quick-thinking. He performed CPR to bring him back from the brink. Thanks to his son's heroics, the older man comes to his feet and is back on his feet. He was whisked to the emergency room, fully conscious and making sense of it all. The biggest twist I found in the story is that his heart's aortic valve is in bad shape, severely narrowed, a condition known as aortic stenosis. After some careful work, we stabilized him and replaced that troublesome aortic valve. Fast forward two years, and he's living life to the fullest.

So, here's the lesson in this heart-pounding story: The shouting and the surge of anger during the argument, along with the sudden stress, stirred up an arrhythmia and even caused a cardiac arrest. The son's knowledge of CPR saved the day, giving his dad a second chance at life. A reminder that in moments of crisis, knowing what to do can be the ultimate lifeline.

In places with medical equipment or Automated External Defibrillators (AEDs), a shock can be given to the person's chest while doing CPR. This is to fix any problems with their heart rhythm and help it beat normally again. But remember, pressing on the chest with CPR is more important than giving a shock. If you have an AED, the correct order is to start with chest compressions, give one shock if needed, and continue with more chest compressions. This cycle can be repeated until the person begins breathing and has a heartbeat again. Usually, about four cycles are done before deciding what to do next, but sometimes, medical professionals might do a few more cycles to give the person the best chance. In a medical environment, experts usually perform five cycles of CPR, which takes around 20 minutes. If the patient fails to recover during this time, it is considered sudden cardiac death. In such cases, determining the exact time frame before declaring a person dead remains a topic of debate. However, the most widely accepted norm defines sudden cardiac death as occurring when a person experiences cardiac arrest and cannot be resuscitated within one hour. This is applicable when someone is being monitored. If a person dies of cardiac arrest without anyone around, it is still considered sudden cardiac death if it happened within 24 hours of them last being seen by someone. This general norm is followed to determine the timeframe for sudden cardiac death.

A 35-year-old guy suddenly finds himself in the grip of excruciating chest pain, and he's drenched in sweat. But it got even scarier – he collapsed. It was a total nightmare. Luckily, his alert friend steps in like a hero, doing CPR and getting him to the nearest hospital in a flash. Something remarkable happened during the ride to the hospital. The guy regained consciousness, and he started breathing normally. It's like he's been given a second chance at life. On arrival, we performed an ECG on his heart, and it told us the story of acute myocardial infarction, the medical term for a heart attack. More specifically, a gnarly type of heart rhythm trouble called VT/VF led to his dramatic collapse, essentially a cardiac arrest.

What saved the day, you ask? Well, it was his friend's knowledge of CPR. That magic trick brought him back from the verge of death. We put a stent in a significant heart artery (LAD). Just two days later, he was back home, recovering.

This is a remarkable tale of a heart attack followed by a heart-stopping arrhythmia-induced cardiac arrest. It teaches us a valuable lesson: CPR and a little electrical shock (DC shock) are like the secret weapons to rescue folks who face a dangerous heart rhythm problem immediately after a heart attack. It's a reminder that knowledge and quick action can be the difference between life and death.

Heart attack mimickers

Certain conditions like aortic dissection (tear in the aorta's inner layer) and pulmonary embolism can mimic heart attack symptoms. **Aortic dissection** patients have severe tearing pain in the back, profuse sweating, and sudden fluctuations in blood pressure. These conditions may be mistaken for a heart attack. Still, they could indicate aortic dissection, where the primary artery(aorta) coming out from the heart has a tear, leading to sudden blood loss from the aorta into the vessel wall and threatening the circulation of vital organs, including coronary circulation as well as leaking of aortic valve (aortic regurgitation). It is also life-threatening in hypertensive, smokers, and Marfan syndrome & other connective tissue diseases.

Pulmonary embolism happens in some predisposed patients. Here, the patient has severe chest discomfort with severe breathlessness. The symptom may mimic a heart attack, but the patient's occluded pulmonary artery is responsible for the sign. It is also a lethal disease and is sometimes missed and underdiagnosed.

Stroke

A stroke occurs when there is a compromise in the circulation to a part of the brain. It is essential to clarify that we use the term "stroke" solely for the brain in medical terminology. In contrast, people sometimes use "heart stroke" and "brain stroke" interchangeably in common language. However, there is no such thing as a "heart stroke." Heart failure, heart attack, and cardiac arrest are different conditions associated with the heart, as we have discussed earlier. Stroke refers explicitly to a brain stroke, which occurs when the brain has compromised blood flow. In medical terminology, we refer to a stroke as a CVA, which stands for Cerebrovascular Accident.

7

CORONARY ARTERY DISEASE (CAD)

"The shattering of a heart when being broken is the loudest quiet ever."

- Carroll Bryant

Cardiovascular disease (CVD) is a group of disorders of the heart and blood vessels, including coronary heart disease, cerebrovascular disease, rheumatic heart disease, and other conditions. They are the leading cause of death globally, taking an estimated 17.9 million lives annually. Over four out of five CVD deaths are due to heart attacks and strokes, and one-third of these deaths occur prematurely in people under 70. In India, for the year 2014, CVDs were reported as the most important causes of death and led to 2.48 million deaths/year comprising deaths from IHD (1.45 million/y), stroke (0.69 million/y), rheumatic heart disease (0.11 million/y) and other CVDs. It is well known that up to a third of cardiovascular deaths can be avoided by proper treatment and control of hypertension, and by addressing this risk factor, we can significantly prevent premature CVD mortality in India.

Coronary Artery Disease (CAD) is the primary classification among the four types of heart diseases. It prevails as the most frequently diagnosed cardiovascular disease among heart patients and is the leading cause of death worldwide. Despite the advancements in modern medicine and procedures that have reduced the mortality rate of CAD, the number of cases continues to surge, resembling a pandemic-like situation.

This chapter delves into comprehending the presentation of Coronary Artery Disease (CAD) which can vary depending on age and comorbidities, along with the medications, procedures, and treatment options treatments available at present. Furthermore, it explores strategies to manage the condition while embracing a fulfilling life, minimizing the risk of its recurrence, and averting other potential heart complications.

Coronary Arteries

Coronary arteries are the vital blood vessels responsible for supplying blood to the heart and ensuring proper functioning. While the heart receives venous blood from all organs and pumps oxygenated blood back to each of them for their functions, it also receives blood separately through two coronary arteries at the beginning of the aorta. The aorta is the primary artery originating from the heart's left ventricle. Interestingly, unlike other arteries supplying organs during systole (when the heart contracts), the two coronary arteries and the heart muscle, or myocardium, operate in a way where the coronary arteries receive blood during diastole (when the heart relaxes). This unique design ensures that while perfusion to other organs occurs during systole, the heart is perfused mostly during diastole.

Two coronary arteries arise from either side (right and left) of the aorta. The left coronary artery further divides into the Left Anterior Descending artery (LAD) and the Left Circumflex artery (LCX), two significant branches of the left coronary artery. We must note that we use terms such as "triple vessel disease"(three-vessel disease) even though we all have only two coronary arteries. The two major branches of the left coronary artery (LAD & LCX) and the right coronary artery are three vessels. However, there are only two coronaries, with the left part dividing into the Left Anterior Descending and Left Circumflex branches.

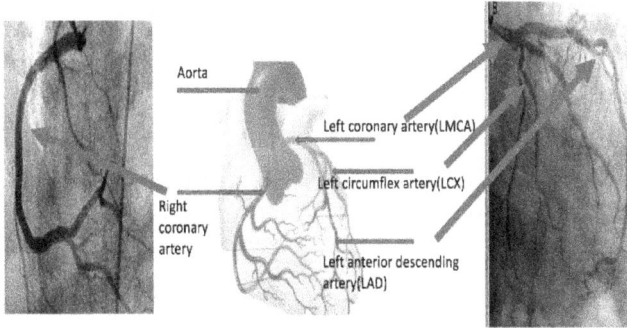

Our heart's unique and robust structure enables it to function continuously and efficiently to keep all bodily systems running smoothly. The circulation must be optimized during the daytime when we are active and at nighttime when we are resting. The coronary artery and its branches are crucial in maintaining continuous and well-perfused heart muscles, allowing the heart to contract and relax effectively day and night.

Atherosclerosis

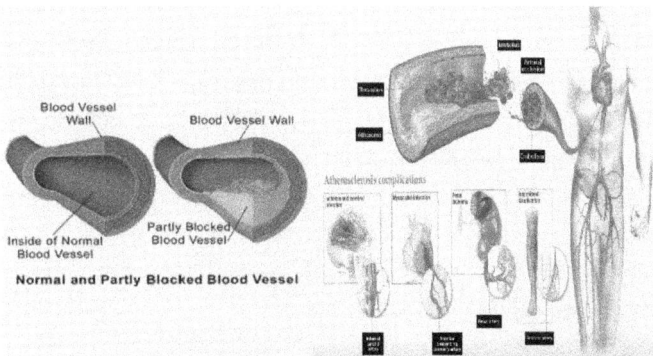

Atherosclerosis and Cardiovascular Disease

As previously mentioned, coronary artery disease (CAD) occurs when a blockage or obstruction inside the coronary arteries reduces or stops blood circulation to the heart. The leading cause of this blockage is Atherosclerosis, a condition that affects various arteries in the body. Atherosclerosis involves the deposition of fats inside the blood vessels, compromising blood flow. When this condition affects the coronary arteries, it leads to CAD.

The inner layer of an artery, the endothelium, consists of endothelial cells, and the open channel inside the vessel is called the lumen. The endothelium becomes dysfunctional and sticky when oxidative injury or inflammation inside the endothelial cells exists. As a result, fat can get deposited inside the artery's wall. This fat is engulfed by residing white blood cells as a protective response, forming foam cells. The abundance of foam cells and spillage of fat into the artery lumen leads to the formation of atherosclerotic plaques.

These fat deposits or plaques grow abluminal initially before crusading into the lumen. Hence, plaque growth has two phases in the timeline. One is negative remodeling, where the vessel area decreases as the plaque narrows the lumen by 40%. The other is positive remodeling, a reparative mechanism where the endothelium tries to prevent the plaque from narrowing the lumen by increasing the vessel size to maintain blood flow. Positive and negative remodeling are undesirable conditions, but positive remodeling can be more dangerous as it can lead to plaque rupture and the formation of clots, causing coronary blockage. You may have heard that a person who has undergone all tests, including angiography, turned out to be normal but developed a heart attack the next day. It is a surprise! In coronary angiography, we look at positive remodeling-induced stenosis (coronary block). However, we should be aware that coronary artery disease is an atherosclerotic manifestation, and negative remodeling (abluminal) takes positive remodeling (luminal narrowing) before. A normal coronary angiography can be deceptive as atherosclerotic plaques, usually not visible in angiography, can turn into unstable plaque at any time and develop total thrombosis of the vessel in which they are located. That's why medical management with lifestyle modification is the first and foremost strategy to prevent heart attacks. It reduces the risk of progression of plaque growth and vulnerability.

Plaques can be classified into two types: soft and hard or calcified. Soft plaques are not easily visible on angiography but are responsible for most heart attacks. They have a fragile upper layer, and when inflamed cells come into contact with blood, clot formation can occur rapidly, leading to severe blockage. This process is unpredictable.

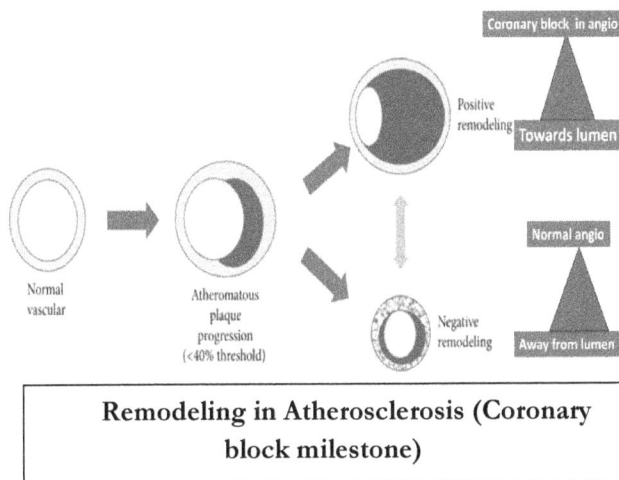

Remodeling in Atherosclerosis (Coronary block milestone)

On the other hand, thick plaques are more stable and can result from better lifestyle modifications and lower oxidative stress levels. Controlling the instability of thin plaques through risk markers can lead to their conversion into thick plaques, which can be cleared by the body's fibers, reducing the risk of plaque rupture and heart attacks.

Research on why and how plaques become inflamed and later rupture has not provided definitive answers. The plaque's destabilization is causing a heart attack, leading to obstruction of blood flow in the major coronary artery. In this abrupt process, a thrombus attaches itself to an area of destabilized plaque. These areas of plaque were not necessarily obstructing to start with and hence may not be visible in coronary angiograms, and that provides an explanation behind the observation that about 50% of all people who have a myocardial infarction (half of which are fatal) do not have symptoms beforehand. The predictability of which thin plaque will rupture remains to be explored, as in-depth research on plaque rupture, stabilization medication, and Atherosclerosis is ongoing. Nevertheless, it is crucial to manage all risk factors to prevent or mitigate the development of CAD.

One of my patients was a 38-year-old guy who's been living a pretty sedentary life, and to add a little drama, there's a history of early heart trouble in his family. So, as a precaution, he went through a bunch of non-invasive heart tests, and his coronary calcium was zero. But he was left scratching his head because his treadmill test (TMT) didn't give a clear answer. He wasn't one to back down, and he wanted to know what was happening with his heart and those pesky blockages. After a chat, I explained that the ultimate way to get the scoop is through a CT angiogram or a coronary angiography, like a heart scan, to check for blockages. So, we did the angiography, and guess what? It was all clear. The guy went home smiling, knowing his blood markers were green and his "gold standard" angiogram was normal. Life was good, or so it seemed. Fast forward just two days, and he's back in our emergency room, in the grips of an acute inferior wall MI (Myocardial Infarction) with his right coronary artery blocked. It was like a lightning bolt out of nowhere. We rushed him into action, performing an emergency angioplasty with a stent. This story carries a crucial message: having a clean bill of health on your coronary angiogram doesn't make you immune to a heart attack, not by a long shot. You see, plaque buildup on the outer layer of arteries can get inflamed and worse overnight, becoming a heart attack. It's a reminder that when you've got risk factors like a sedentary lifestyle and a family history of heart disease, you can't afford to take it lightly, even if your angiogram looks hunky-dory. Lifestyle changes and medications are your best friends, even without apparent blockages. In this guy's case, those risk factors were real troublemakers.

Spectrum of Coronary Artery Disease

Coronary Artery Disease (CAD) is classified into two types: Acute Coronary Syndrome and Chronic Coronary Syndrome. Acute Coronary Syndrome(ACS) refers to emergency heart attacks, while Chronic Coronary Syndrome is a gradually progressive coronary artery narrowing presenting with stable angina symptoms. Here, a patient can sometimes have a totally occluded coronary artery with relatively few symptoms, which is paradoxical to our expectations. As with any slowly progressive disease, as in chronic CAD, our body responds to counter the challenge by taking action against it. The growth of collateral circulation may only be visible if its size is above the resolution of a coronary angiogram, which is 500 microns. They feed the blocked artery's territory when the block grows slowly.

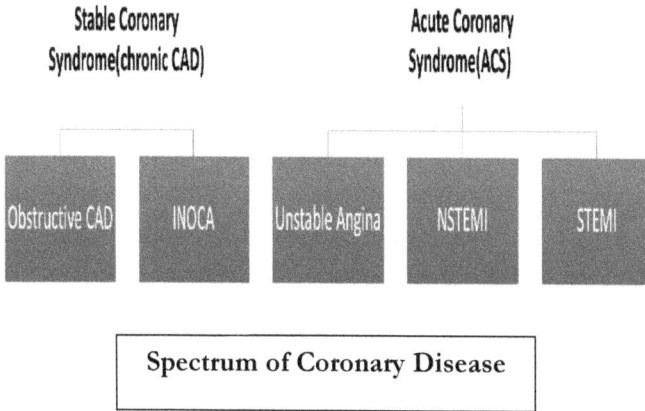

Stable Coronary Syndrome(chronic CAD)   **Acute Coronary Syndrome(ACS)**

| Obstructive CAD | INOCA | Unstable Angina | NSTEMI | STEMI |

Spectrum of Coronary Disease

Acute Coronary Syndrome

Acute Coronary Syndrome is classified into three variants depending on ECG and blood markers: ST Elevation MI (STEMI), Non-ST Elevation MI (NSTEMI), and Unstable Angina. A heart attack is a myocardial infarction(MI) in medical terminology.

ST Elevation MI (STEMI)- In ST Elevation MI, a specific segment of the Electrocardiogram (ECG) shows the classical changes called displacement of the ST segment, which establishes the diagnosis and gives a clue about the blocked artery. We call it the culprit artery. The STEMI is a more severe type of heart attack with serious complications due to total blockage of one or more primary coronary arteries, leading to the death of the heart muscle (called infarction) that is not receiving adequate blood flow. The most accessible tool to detect is ECG, which reflects typical changes when a heart attack is ongoing. Therefore, ECG is a crucial tool in investigating a heart attack, and it should be performed as early as possible if the patient is experiencing chest pain. Patients who cannot reach a cardiologist immediately should go to the nearest center for an ECG. Comparing the current ECG with a previous one when the patient was normal can provide valuable information regarding this medical emergency.

For patients with **ST Elevation MI,** we offer two immediate treatment options. The preferred and best option is primary Angioplasty, also called primary PCI (percutaneous cardiac intervention), where a procedure is performed to clear the blockage in the coronary artery. However, Thrombolysis is performed as an alternative in medical centers not equipped with a cardiac CATH laboratory (CATHLAB) facility. Thrombolysis has certain limitations, including time constraints, contraindications, and success rate, which depend on two critical factors. The time we are doing Thrombolysis from the onset of heart attack and the drug we use for Thrombolysis. It works very well in the golden hour (1 hour of myocardial infarction/heart attack), but maximum, it can be given up to 12 hours after a heart attack.

Moving on to **Non-ST Elevation MI**, the ECG does not show classical ST-segment elevation in this condition, but blood markers like CK-MB and Trop T may be positive. The ECG may also offer other findings indicating a partial blockage in a coronary artery. Non-ST Elevation MI is considered a milder state than STEMI, but still, it is a heart attack. The treatment for NSTEMI can vary from patient to patient, ranging from medications to Angioplasty or bypass surgery. Here, *thrombolysis* (clot-dissolving medication) plays no role, specifically for patients with STEMI only.

Unstable Angina - The third variant of Acute CAD is called Unstable Angina. Stable angina refers to experiencing cardiac chest pain during a particular activity or fixed threshold, and it falls under Chronic CAD. However, this stable angina can progress to Unstable Angina, which again a cardiac emergency. Unstable angina is characterized by anginal chest pain at rest or increasing frequency or reducing the threshold for the onset of angina when the patient cannot perform activities they could normally do. For example, suppose a person used to walk 500 meters daily before he experienced any anginal pain, but now he experiences the same at around 200 meters. In that case, it is considered a new onset of angina and marks instability of previously stable CAD. Unstable angina often results from a partial blockage of a coronary artery. It is the starting point that can lead to NSTEMI and, if untreated, can evolve into STEMI, where the blood circulation to a particular part of the heart muscle is completely blocked.

Challenges in chest pain -Emotion to Legal

Chest pain is sometimes very challenging to establish or rule out cardiac emergency, mainly when your baseline ECG is abnormal or unavailable. In cases with no past ECG available, blood markers such as Trop T, Trop I, or CPK-MB indicate ischemia (lack of blood flow to the heart). However, it takes time for these markers to reach a threshold for a positive or negative result, usually around 6-12 hours. Other investigations may also be performed to assess the situation further. Currently, 0/1 and 0/2 protocols with high-sensitivity troponin rule out acute coronary syndrome. When the patient reports, the hs-Troponin level and 1 or 2 hrs level can establish or rule out ACS.

Chest pain is a complaint that can be challenging to diagnose as a heart attack. Even if the ECG does not show significant abnormalities, ruling out a heart attack without further investigations is impossible, especially if the patient is experiencing ongoing chest pain. This uncertainty in diagnosis has been utilized by criminals and corrupt politicians, mainly when they are about to be arrested. The challenges of chest pain diagnosis as heart attack allow avoiding being arrested for judicial inquiry and buying time to escape from jail custody and stay in a comfortable hospital setting for at least 24 hours or more.

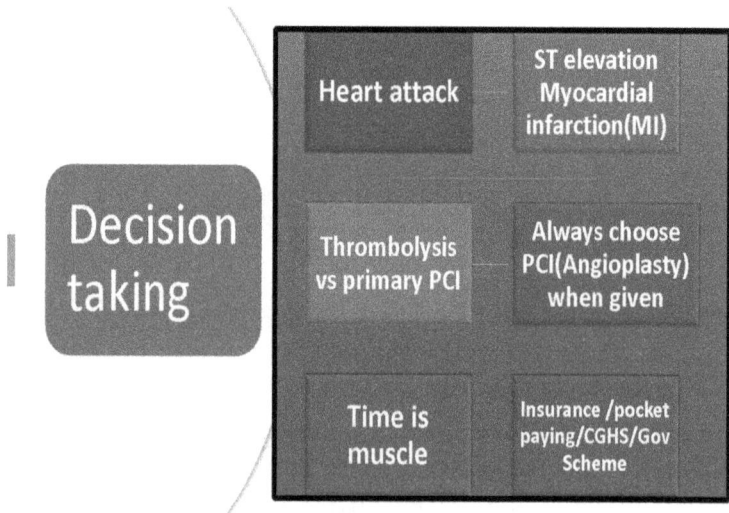

Decision taking	Heart attack	ST elevation Myocardial infarction(MI)
	Thrombolysis vs primary PCI	Always choose PCI(Angioplasty) when given
	Time is muscle	Insurance /pocket paying/CGHS/Gov Scheme

In summary, all three types, including unstable angina, non-ST elevation, and ST elevation MI, share the common problem of compromised blood circulation. While ST elevation MI can be diagnosed by observing the ST elevation on the ECG, the other two types require differentiation based on raised blood marker levels like Trop T and CK-MB.

👤 **Reduce mental tension**

🏃 **Reduce physical activity of patient**

✏ **Reach early hospital-confirmation and treatment**

📍 **Rush to the nearest center with facility as early as possible**

🩺 **Never chase the center/doctor if it is far away**

> **During Heart Attack- Reduce Harm First (Salvage Myocardium)**

Treatments & Medicines for Acute CAD (Heart Attack)

Two types of treatments are initiated when a person arrives at the hospital after experiencing a heart attack. The key is initial medication, including blood thinners, anti-cholesterol drugs, and clot-dissolving medicines. The immediate treatment involves administering a loading dose of medicines like Aspirin, Blood thinners, Statins (Anti-cholesterol drugs), and anticoagulants like Heparin. Sorbitrate or Nitrates may also be placed under the tongue to improve coronary circulation. These preventive medicines are often given upon arrival at the hospital. Once a patient is diagnosed with myocardial infarction heart attack through ECG and is experiencing ongoing chest pain, the window period for treatment to minimize further heart damage is very important. The sooner we treat, the better the heart's functioning will be. Delaying treatment results in more muscle power loss for the heart. Patients sometimes contemplate the best treatment option among Thrombolysis versus Angioplasty. However, the longer the decision-making process takes, the more strength the heart muscles are lost, possibly leading to irreversible heart failure. Accepting the disease, deciding early, and promptly moving forward with treatment is crucial. It is essential to know that Primary Angioplasty (also called Primary PCI) is the best treatment for all heart attack (myocardial infarction), and it score above Thrombolysis in most situation.

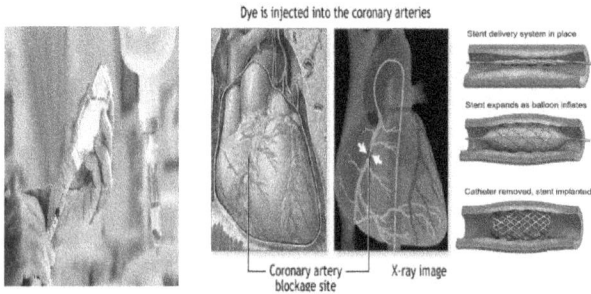

Dye is injected into the coronary arteries

Stent delivery system in place

Stent expands as balloon inflates

Catheter removed, stent implanted

Coronary artery blockage site — X-ray image

Making choice between Thrombolysis vs. Primary Angioplasty during Heart Attack

Primary PCI & Balloon Angioplasty

Angioplasty or PCI (Percutaneous Coronary Intervention) is a minimally invasive procedure that offers ease of execution and faster patient recovery. In cases where the medical facility lacks a Cath Lab for Angioplasty, Facilitated PCI can be considered, where fibrinolytic therapy is used to stabilize the patient while arranging transport to a primary PCI facility for the angioplasty procedure and postoperative monitoring. This perioperative approach is crucial in managing acute coronary syndrome, which demands immediate attention.

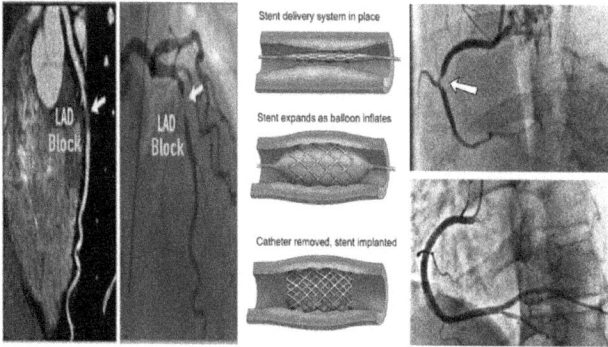

> **Coronary Block (Stenosis)- Coronary Angioplasty and Stenting**

During Angioplasty, a cardiologist inserts catheters through the leg artery (femoral approach) or hand artery (radial approach) and injects dye to identify the affected coronary artery, also called the culprit artery. Initially, we pass wire to cross the blocked lesion, followed by a wire balloon to plaster the clot/ thrombus to the artery wall, which has occluded the artery and established the coronary circulation. It is followed by the deployment of the stent, a metallic scaffold that prevents occlusion of the coronary artery in the block's location that underwent ballooning. While metal stents were previously utilized, modern drug-coated stents consist of a mesh-like metal stent coated with drugs that reduce the risk of restenosis over time. Angioplasty and stenting in the setting of myocardial infarction is called primary PCI, now considered the gold standard for treating heart attacks or Acute Coronary Syndrome, surpassing Thrombolysis in efficacy.

Thrombolysis

Thrombolysis is vital when the ECG confirms CAD with ST-elevation MI(STEMI). This treatment is limited to the first 12 hours after chest pain or angina onset. Due to economic reasons and availability constraints, Thrombolysis can be a suitable alternative to Angioplasty in selected patients.

In Thrombolysis, we attempt to dissolve the thrombus by administering medicine intravenously. There are two types of Thrombolysis based on the method and substance used – either through transfusion or a bolus. This method only applies within the *first 12 hours* of a Heart Attack and *only for ST Elevation Myocardial Infarction (STEMI)*. For cases where the ECG does not show ST elevations, such as unstable angina or non-ST elevation MI (NSTEMI), which are also classified as acute coronary syndromes, Thrombolysis is not employed. Therefore, thrombolysis is an option only for STEMI within 12 hours.

Complication and course of Heart Attack

During a heart attack, various subsequent events can occur in the heart, from rhythm disorders to valve dysfunction. The first few hours after a heart attack are considered the most vulnerable period for critical rhythm disorders. If they happen, the episodes of killer rhythm disorders like ventricular tachycardia and ventricular fibrillation can be fatal. They are responsible for most of the sudden death after a heart attack at home or during transit to the hospital.

Some patients develop issues related to normal current flow between the upper and lower chambers, called AV conduction disorder. It happens more in specific territories, such as the right coronary artery or left circumflex territory block, which supplies the crucial AV node(heart transmitter). If the AV node is compromised, the heart's beating can slow down, leading to symptoms like giddiness syncope and can progress to cardiac arrest and death if not corrected by external cardiac pacing. It can also lead to valvular dysfunction, most commonly of the mitral valve, which may leak, causing backflow, a condition known as *mitral regurgitation*. Additionally, the heart can develop holes due to the rupture of its wall or the septum separating the left and right lower chamber (ventricle). This is called Myocardial Rupture or Ventricular

Septal Rupture. These mechanical complications can develop during the first few days, mostly in reporting cases of heart attack (those who have a heart attack ongoing for many hours or days before reaching the hospital) or non-revascularized heart attacks. Electrical complications may lead to cardiac arrest and death. In contrast, mechanical complications can surprise us, causing a sudden drop in blood pressure, sudden severe breathlessness, and potentially leading to cardiac arrest that can progress to death.

Heart attacks can lead to critical situations from which recovery becomes challenging. It is essential to monitor heart attack patients closely for a few days. Another potential complication during a heart attack is Pericarditis. In Pericarditis, the patient experiences chest pain, which is non-angina, even though it originates from the heart. It has the characteristics of *pleurisy*, which means it increases deep inspiration and coughing. It is not due to vascular compromise; it is caused by inflammation in and around the heart. Unlike mechanical or electrical complications, Pericarditis generally has a fair prognosis. Patients with Pericarditis may have a fever and experience more pain when coughing or changing their posture. This condition usually occurs with a severe heart attack (large area myocardial infarct) and in those who come late after the onset of a heart attack.

Sometimes, the patient may experience heart failure during a heart attack, where the heart fails to pump enough blood to supply all other organs effectively. This situation is referred to as cardiogenic shock. As a result of reduced blood flow and hypotension, perfusion to the brain, kidneys, or limbs is impaired, which can become cold and clammy. The patient may develop *oliguria* (decreased urine output) or *anuria* (no urine output). Cardiogenic shock is a grave condition in heart attack, and the survival and recovery chances drop to 50-50 chance. Therefore, cardiogenic shock is considered one of the deadly complications during a heart attack.

Chronic Coronary Artery Disease

Chronic Coronary Syndrome is when someone has a heart problem that's been there for a while. They might have already had treatment like getting a stent or having surgery to fix it, or they could take medicine to help with chest pain and slow the heart problem from worsening. Let us be clear that *any new onset of anginal chest pain or anginal chest pain at rest* should be considered an acute coronary syndrome or heart attack and investigated & treated accordingly. It later comes under the umbrella of Chronic CAD when there is no clinical progression of the disease, and complaints are relieved on medication. Some patients may have angina for a prolonged period before coming to medical attention. It may be two to three years, occurring during specific physical activities such as walking or running after a particular distance. If left untreated, Chronic CAD can be punctuated with episodes of ACS needing hospitalization and treatment. Patients in this category may be in the early stages of CAD or experiencing a recurrence of CAD after previously having a heart attack and receiving medication with or without a stent. Symptoms may be present, but sometimes, patients can be asymptomatic and unaware of the condition. Experienced doctors can diagnose Chronic CAD through clinical history before confirming it through physical examinations and investigations.

Symptoms of coronary circulation issues, such as angina and breathlessness, are vital aspects of the clinical diagnosis. Typically, these symptoms are associated with physical activity, with the pain occurring during exertion and subsiding during rest. When this pattern is consistently observed, it is known as stable angina or angina pectoris. Chronic CAD and Acute coronary syndrome (heart attack) are usually present with Angina Pectoris with or without breathlessness. The differentiation between acute and chronic is vital. Medical management is typically preferred over intervention for Chronic CAD, and interventions (coronary angiography, Angioplasty, coronary bypass grafting) are done when medical management does not relieve the complaint or *provide a quick-fix solution* to the complaint of heart symptoms related to circulation. In acute coronary syndrome, STEMI intervention (primary Angioplasty and stenting) is preferred and more rewarding than conservative medical management. Both are followed by lifelong medication, including blood thinners and cholesterol-lowering drugs, which are crucial for managing these diseases. Patients need to follow a heart-healthy diet and address risk factors proactively. Accepting the disease and actively participating in the treatment are vital aspects of living harmoniously with these conditions.

How to diagnose Coronary Block?

During cardiac evaluation, patients can have baseline abnormalities ECG or findings of a previous heart attack. Most of the time, ECG are normal in patients with chronic CAD. An Echocardiography (Echo) adds information regarding heart pumping power reflected as cardiac ejection fraction. It detects parts of the heart muscle that are not contracting normally, called regional wall motion abnormality *(RWMA)*. But again, it can also be normal, even in chronic CAD. If the diagnosis remains uncertain after preliminary symptoms, ECG, echo tests, CT coronary artery calcium scoring (CAC score), and CT coronary angiography (CTCA) are noninvasive options. CAC Score measures calcified plaque in the coronary arteries, while CTCA provides detailed imaging of any coronary circulation blocks. In some patients, nuclear perfusion scanning and TMT (Treadmill Test) are other noninvasive methods for predicting coronary artery disease. A Dobutamine Stress Evaluation (DSE) is an alternative when the patient cannot walk for TMT. We administer drugs like dobutamine, creating controlled stress on the heart by increasing heart rate and contractility, followed by an echocardiogram to look for discrepancies in muscle contraction with increased heart rate in a controlled environment. That explains how muscle contraction is compromised during stress due to coronary perfusion defects. Nuclear Scanning is another investigation using a radio-nucleotide to assess blood circulation. If none of the noninvasive tests provide a clear picture of the blockage, the final and still gold standard investigation is Coronary Angiography, a minimally invasive procedure. This involves injecting a radiocontrast(dye) into the coronary artery by a catheter placed at its mouth (ostium) and visualizing the coronary blood flow and stenosis (block) in any of the artery or its branch in real-time an X-ray machine called a Cath Lab. This diagnostic procedure is called coronary angiogram and is done by radial(hand) or femoral(leg) route.

Treatment for chronic CAD

Treatment for CAD involves various medications, including antiplatelet drugs, Statins (cholesterol-lowering medications), Beta blockers, and ACE inhibitors. Medicines like nicorandil, trimetazidine, or ranolazine may be prescribed to improve blood circulation further. Regardless of whether the condition is Chronic CAD de novo or disease after a heart attack (ACS), which was treated with coronary Revascularization by stenting the culprit's vessel, coronary artery disease is *a lifelong disease* and part of a generalized disease called Atherosclerosis. It is *a localized manifestation of generalized disease*, and it is essential to appreciate that *stenting is the localized fixing* of the problem of block in index location. Still, the disease is smoldering, and generalized vascular inflammation is ongoing.

Hence, treatment primarily involves medication, lifestyle modifications, and risk management throughout life. Coronary angiography provides the necessary information to plan further treatment if medications prove ineffective and symptoms persist or recur in chronic CAD.

It is crucial to profile the patient over some time and consider their medical history before resorting to invasive procedures like angiography. For instance, if a patient with hypertension and diabetes experiences chest pain or heaviness while walking a certain distance but does not have any time at rest and acute finding of heart attack (ECG, Trop T/I, and echogram are normal), it could be indicative of compromised circulation and CAD. Still, other factors, such as anemia (low HB) and essential evaluations, should be checked before angiography to rule out alternative causes. Assessing each patient's condition carefully and considering medical management before proceeding with invasive procedures is necessary. The goal is to find the most suitable and effective treatment approach for managing CAD and ensuring patient outcomes.

Coronary Revascularization in chronic CAD- the Why, When, How, Who of cardiac revascularization

The Coronary Revascularization is the final solution of significant coronary artery disease with symptoms of angina. There are two types- minimally invasive procedures done by interventional cardiologists called coronary Angioplasty and stenting, and the second method is coronary artery bypass surgery, which is an open-heart surgery done by a cardiothoracic surgeon, also called a CTVS surgeon.

WHY should revascularization be done?

Blood thinners(antiplatelets), cholesterol-lowering medicines, antihypertensive, antidiabetic, and other supportive medications, including nitrates, are commonly prescribed to manage the condition medically (noninvasive conservative management). With proper medication, diet, and lifestyle modifications, patients may experience improved health and develop collateral circulation in the compromised coronary territory, reducing the need for invasive cardiac interventions (coronary angiography, Angioplasty, and stenting or CABG). Sometimes, even after doing this above-mentioned medical management, quality of life remains compromised with recurrent angina and breathlessness. Hence, cardiac intervention (Revascularization by doing stenting or CABG) is the best solution.

WHEN should Revascularization be done?

With proper medications, diet, and lifestyle modifications, patients complain of compromised coronary territory, presenting as angina and breathlessness. If it doesn't subside, invasive cardiac interventions (coronary angiography followed by coronary Angioplasty with stenting or CABG) are the final resort in cases of chronic CAD. It is a quick-fix solution for the coronary circulatory compromise and the fear surrounding the course of coronary block. Cardiac intervention (Revascularization by stenting or CABG) is the best solution when medical management fails.

HOW should Revascularization be done?

Medical management includes drugs that modify either cardiac metabolism or augment coronary circulation. It also reduces vascular inflammation(Atherosclerosis). Hence, it should not be stopped *at any time* in managing coronary artery disease. However, the local solution of advanced coronary compromise, which doesn't yield to medical management, is local intervention by coronary Angioplasty and stenting. Coronary artery bypass grafting (CABG) is a local modification of coronary circulation by adding more conduits between the aorta and coronary artery(venous conduit) or adding chest vessel artery(arterial conduits-LIMA, RIMA, BIMA) to coronary circulation.

CABG augments the compromised circulation by bypassing the blocked coronary location through the arterial or venous conduits.

WHO should opt for Revascularization?

Any coronary blockage in LAD, LCX, or RCA that exceeds 70% of the artery's diameter, Angioplasty, and stenting or bypass surgery becomes necessary if the patients remain symptomatic on medical management. Any branch of the artery mentioned above (LAD,

LCX, RCA) more than 2.5mm in diameter should be considered for Revascularization. In the LMCA(left main coronary artery), which later on divides and becomes LAD and LCX, the threshold for intervention is more than 50% stenosis of diameter, unlike 75% of the above vessels(LAD, LCX, RCA), where we do an intervention. The decision on whether to opt for stenting or bypass depends on many factors like the location, anatomy, severity of block, and associated comorbidity. In specific situations like Left Main Coronary Artery Disease (LMCA), Proximal LAD (Left Anterior Descending), or Bifurcation Blockage, CABG surgery may be favored over stenting, especially in diabetic patients.

Coronary Artery Bypass (CABG) Surgery

In CABG surgery, as the name suggests, we create an alternative circulation path to bypass the blocked artery, unlike Angioplasty, where we use a stent to open the blockage. During bypass surgery, a portion of a vessel or conduit is taken from another part of the patient's body to create the bypass route. There are two methods of bypass surgery - arterial graft and venous graft - where we use either an arterial conduit or a venous conduit, respectively, as the bypassing path.

An arterial graft involves using the arterial vessels as conduits and, most commonly, the Left and right internal mammary arteries called LIMA and RIMA, respectively, which supply the chest wall and have been observed to have good longevity without blockage after being used for the bypass. On the other hand, venous grafts mainly involve taking veins from the vascular part of the leg, such as the great saphenous vein, which is relatively large and has a bit shorter longevity compared to arterial grafts.

During the bypass surgery, the selected arterial or venous conduit is dissected, cleaned, and used to connect from the aorta to the later part of the artery after the coronary blockage. This way, the old artery continues to supply blood up to the blockage while the new bypass nourishes the heart muscle beyond the blockage, ensuring complete nourishment of the heart muscle.

Remember that Atherosclerosis is a lifelong disease, and the bypassed conduits are a local augmentation of blood flow in the heart circulation. However, by maintaining an active lifestyle and taking good care of health with medicines, diet, and exercises, one can develop *alternative circulations (collateral circulation)* that can compensate for such blockages over time.

Unlike Angioplasty and stenting, which a cardiologist performs is less invasive and shorter hospital stay, coronary artery bypass graft (CABG) surgery is a fully invasive open-heart procedure and is performed by a cardiothoracic surgeon. Therefore, the surgeon's experience and expertise are critical to the procedure's success.

EECP - An alternative to stenting or CABG

In cases where patients cannot undergo Angioplasty or bypass surgery or are unwilling to undergo any invasive revascularization procedure due to increased life risk, enhanced external counterpulsation (EECP) therapy may be considered. It is a non-invasive treatment to reduce the frequency and intensity of angina episodes. It is administered through three external inflatable cuffs applied around the lower legs, upper legs, and buttocks. These cuffs provide graded pressure synchronized with the cardiac cycle to lower limbs to improve blood flow in the heart by giving stimulus for collateral circulation. A different number of sessions are needed to alleviate the symptoms of angina through this noninvasive coronary circulation augmentation.

Myths and facts of Chronic CAD

Chronic CAD is a stable but slowly progressing heart disease that, if left untreated, can lead to Acute coronary syndrome and heart failure. Patients with CAD must adhere to their treatment plan, make lifestyle modifications, and actively manage their risk factors to improve their long-term prognosis and overall quality of life.

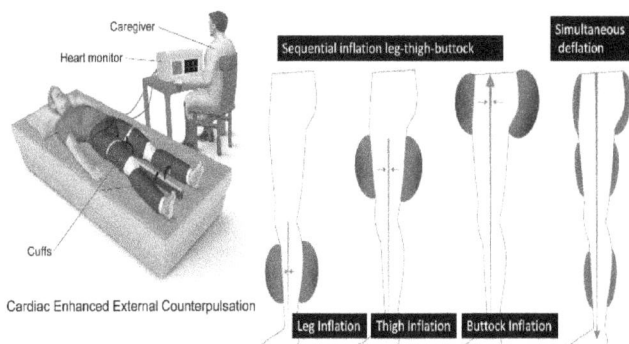

Caregiver
Heart monitor
Sequential inflation leg-thigh-buttock
Simultaneous deflation
Cuffs
Cardiac Enhanced External Counterpulsation
Leg Inflation | Thigh Inflation | Buttock Inflation

Enhanced external counter pulsation (ECCP)

Treadmill Test (TMT)

The routine TMT after coronary intervention should be discouraged and has already been removed from the recent cardiac authority guidelines (ACC and ESC). There is a tendency to perform coronary angiography routinely after coronary stenting or CABG, even if the patient is not having complaints. Sometimes, the patient needs to know about the stent status and the progression of earlier blocks, which were non-obstructive (less than 50% stenosis), and many times, a cardiologist does a routine angiogram even though the patient has no complaints. It is not advisable to undergo and objectify the coronary block status.

Course of Coronary Block and Rule of 70 %

All patients of chronic CAD with symptomatic angina, coronary Angioplasty, and stenting or CABG are recommended after an initial attempt at medical management. Suppose the patient does not respond adequately to medication. In that case, a coronary angiogram should be conducted. Suppose coronary blockages (stenosis) exceed 70%, except for LMCA, where it is 50% or above. In that case, it is considered significant and should be planned for Angioplasty with stenting to alleviate the symptoms of angina.

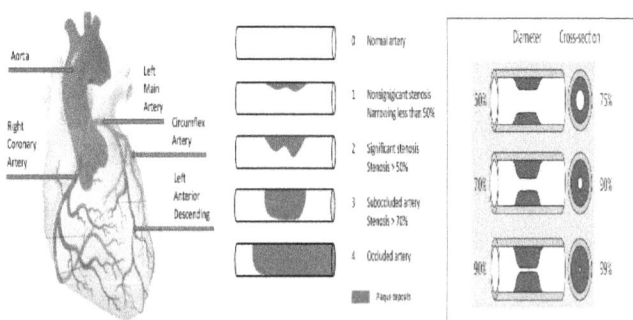

Coronary Block- Diameter Occlusion versus Cross section Occlusion

Patients often have a coronary angiogram done, and disease is present in all three vessels but not significant for Revascularization. *Block of less than 70 % is always treated medically* on drug and lifestyle modification. Patients often fear that these nonsignificant blocks will result in heart attacks and consent to undergo Angioplasty, which is neither correct nor scientifically beneficial. Let us be clear that during angiography, we are having a glimpse of coronary artery and obstruction, if any, in that time frame. Any obstruction less than 70% in diameter only needs medicine to retard progression and stabilize the plaque milieu to prevent heart attack (acute coronary syndrome). It has *never been proven* that stenting or CABG will prevent heart attack in this scenario. Even when it is more than 70% stenosis, the premises for stenting or Revascularization are for relieving symptoms of angina and breathlessness and improving quality of life. The association of survival benefits for patients or prevention of heart attack by Revascularization over medical management has already been questioned in many trials. These trials (COURAGE, BARI-2D, ORBITA, ISCHEMIA) are randomized trials and established that Revascularization by any means, either stenting or CABG, has never reduced heart attack or prolonged longevity by any means. Good medical management is still the sheet anchor treatment for chronic CAD. The bias for the cardiac intervention of all short of a coronary block, particularly in the chronic CAD subset, is more a therapeutic overtreatment than its impact on disease per se, mainly when the patient is asymptomatic on medication. No doubt, the patient feels better, and the fear factor dissolves after the intervention, and it has been well shown in the ORBITA trial (only a sham trial done to show the placebo effect of the stent on angina).

ORBITA Trial
The Lancet Volume 391, p31–40, 6 January 2018

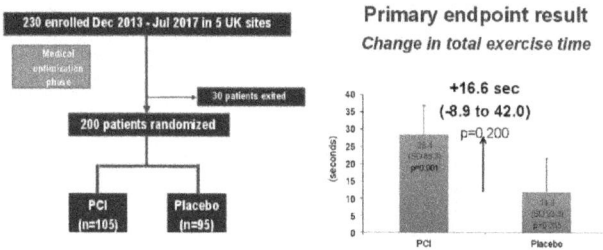

230 enrolled Dec 2013 - Jul 2017 in 5 UK sites

Medical optimization phase

30 patients exited

200 patients randomized

PCI (n=105)   Placebo (n=95)

Primary endpoint result
Change in total exercise time

+16.6 sec
(-8.9 to 42.0)
p=0.200

ORBITA TRIAL- Block Open with Stent vs. No Stenting- SHAM Trial

It is difficult for cardiologists to answer which block will turn into a heart attack. A patient with no obstruction in a routine coronary angiogram (normal Angio) can develop a heart attack even on the day of discharge. A heart attack is more like an accident in which one or other coronary artery can get blocked suddenly and present angina at rest. As accidents happen more on particular roads than others, the same is true with heart attacks. Some individuals who have more risk factors will have more propensity to have heart attacks, while some will have less. Nobody can claim that he has zero risk of heart attack even after doing every possible investigation available on the globe.

Four landmark trial (COURAGE, BARI2D, ORBITA, ISCHEMIA) in past two decades has shown, time and again that in the setting of contemporary GDMT(guideline-directed medical treatment) versus coronary intervention(revascularization) in stable coronary artery disease patients—even those with moderate to severe ischemia and extensive CAD —does **not prolong life or reduce MI** but provide relief from angina especially in patients with daily to weekly angina.

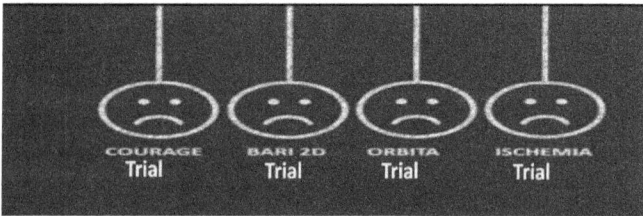

A partially blocked coronary artery (less than 50%) to a normal coronary artery can be the seat of this. It is a change in the local milieu in a particular location in the culprit coronary artery, which inhabits "soft plaques." The changes in this plaque, uncontrolled by normal body homeostasis, are responsible for total artery thrombosis and heart attack. Why did it happen? And when will it happen in that particular location? Medical science has no answer but many hypotheses that finally settle at localized inflammation in plaque culminating into thrombosis of the culprit coronary artery.

Reversal of Coronary Block

Block in coronary artery due to Atherosclerosis is mostly a *one-way gear (only forward, no reverse gear)* except for the thrombus(clot) occlusion. It takes years to a decade to become a significant block. The smoldering inflammation of Atherosclerosis grows abluminal (away from the lumen, which means toward the wall), initially followed by luminal encroachment called positive remodeling. Our body's local homeostasis and reparative mechanism are always on task to control its growth; hence, it takes decades to grow except for thrombus formation at the local side, leading to total occlusion and heart attack. Medical management only decelerates the rate of progression of this Atherosclerosis. So far, we have *no medication to reverse* it, but medication sometimes reduces the block size (stenosis percentage) by reducing the fat core. A full-blown calcified block *neither reduces nor recedes* by any medication. Many claims have been misfeeded in the public domain, showing that drugs or intravenous drug solutions are used to clean the artery and remove blocks. These are false information, and no scientific data supports those practices.

Fallacy regarding coronary artery Calcium (CAC) Scoring

Calcium scoring has gained popularity in recent years. However, it is essential to understand that calcium scoring is an indirect marker of Coronary Artery Disease (CAD), where calcification occurs in the arteries due to plaque calcification. A higher calcium score indicates a more significant disease burden and possible blockage in the arteries. CAC scoring is used for detecting and quantifying calcific coronary Atherosclerosis, but it misses noncalcified coronary atherosclerotic plaque, plaque features, and coronary block; hence, it should not be used to evaluate *symptomatic* patients. It is essential to understand that CAC sore is recommended only for primary prevention decision-making in *asymptomatic* adults who are older than 40 years. In a study, about 58% of patients younger than 40 years and with zero CAC score were found to have obstructive CAD means coronary block more than 50%.

While calcium scoring can help identify the presence or absence of calcified CAD, it cannot predict whether a patient will develop a medical emergency, such as a heart attack, over a specific period. It is crucial to recognize that CT Angiography and Calcium Scoring are diagnostic tools used to confirm the presence of CAD rather than predictive tools for future medical emergencies.

Using these tests routinely for general risk classification in all patients may not be appropriate. The decision to utilize calcium scoring and CT Angiography should be made on a case-by-case basis, considering the patient's clinical presentation, medical history, and risk factors. The primary goal of these tests is to confirm the presence of CAD and guide the appropriate treatment approach, such as starting statin therapy, rather than predicting future medical events.

Other Unusual conditions of CAD

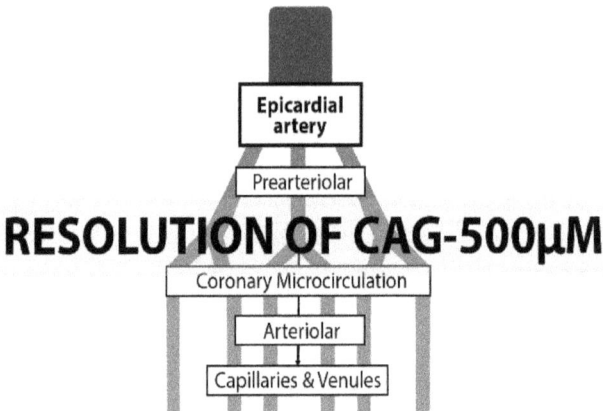

Epicardial artery

Prearteriolar

RESOLUTION OF CAG-500μM

Coronary Microcirculation

Arteriolar

Capillaries & Venules

Coronary Angiogram Resolution (Something is still Hidden)

Ischemia with non-obstructive coronary arteries (INOCA)-The coronary artery disease (CAD) diagnosis typically involves a Coronary angiogram, which provides a comprehensive view of the coronary arteries and any blockages present. However, there are instances where patients may display typical CAD symptoms, but their angiogram results appear normal. This condition is known as myocardial infarction with non-obstructive coronary artery disease (MINOCA), where the major coronary arteries show no signs of illness, but the smaller vessels, called microvessels, may be affected, compromising circulation. This condition is referred to as Microvascular Angina. Although these patients are usually female and experience typical angina during physical activity like walking, they are generally asymptomatic at rest. *A strong-willed 45-year-old woman found herself in the hospital, clutching her chest in agony. Her ECG, the heartbeat of her heart's story, revealed something alarming – Acute Coronary Syndrome (ACS). You might wonder what brought her to this harrowing point in her life.*

It all started with a heart-wrenching piece of news – the accidental death of her beloved father. Imagine the shock, the sadness, and the overwhelming grief she must have felt. To make matters even more complex, she was a divorcee, carrying the weight of single parenthood. Now, when the medical team conducted an angiography, the results left them puzzled. Her coronary arteries, the usual suspects in heart trouble, were fine. It was as if they were looking at a clean slate. However, when they turned their attention to her heart's echo, they discovered something alarming – severe pump failure.

You see, this is a classic case of what we call "broken heart syndrome." It's not just a poetic phrase; it's an actual medical condition. This woman's heart, heavy with grief and burdened by life's challenges, had taken a toll on her. It is a stark reminder that our emotional well-being can profoundly affect our physical health, sometimes leading to unexpected medical mysteries like this one.

As these compromised micro-vessels are not visible on the angiogram (due to their size being below 500 micrometers), further intervention or procedures are not generally recommended. Instead, the treatment involves medications, lifestyle modifications, dietary changes, and regular exercise.

Myocardial Bridge

Another unique condition affecting coronary arteries is the presence of a "coronary bridge." This condition, resulting from a congenital anomaly, occurs when a coronary artery that should run above the muscle is instead located within the muscle. When the heart muscle contracts vigorously, it may compress the artery and compromise blood flow. However, the angiogram may appear to reveal a normal caliber of the coronary artery. For this condition, the primary approach is non-interventional, with medications being the preferred treatment. Sometimes, a stent may be considered, but this option is approached cautiously to avoid compromising future surgical procedures. If conservative treatments fail to address the condition, microsurgery may be performed to free the artery by removing a portion of the surrounding muscle.

In other words, while Coronary Angiography remains the gold standard for diagnosing CAD, specific situations like Microvascular Angina and coronary bridges may reveal normal angiogram even in severe symptoms of angina. Medical management, including medications and lifestyle changes, is the preferred course of action for such cases. When necessary, microsurgery may be employed to address severe conditions with coronary bridges. These cases highlight the complexity of diagnosing and treating CAD, requiring a tailored approach to each patient's unique circumstances.

Other Vascular Diseases like CAD

Indeed, Coronary Artery Disease (CAD) is a critical manifestation of Atherosclerosis, a vascular disease that can affect various arteries in the body. Atherosclerosis can lead to other serious conditions depending on the arteries involved:

Peripheral Vascular Disease (PVD): In PVD, arteries in the lower or upper limbs develop clots or blockages, leading to compromised blood flow to the limb. A sudden onset block occluding the supplying territory of the limb can present with sudden pain in the limb with tingling, numbness, and weakness. If left untreated, acute limb ischemia can occur, which may result in gangrene (death of tissue).

Treatment for PVD is similar to CAD, involving lifestyle modifications such as quitting smoking and taking disease-modifying drugs like blood thinners and cholesterol-lowering medications to slow disease progression. These medications will likely be lifelong, considering atherosclerosis is the underlying cause. Stenting or vascular bypass surgery around the blocked artery may be necessary in acute or emergency.

Cerebrovascular Disease: When Atherosclerosis affects the cerebral arteries that supply blood to the brain, it can lead to cerebrovascular disease. This condition may cause various symptoms related to the brain before significantly affecting brain function. The treatment approach for cerebrovascular disease also involves medical management and intervention as needed.

Renovascular Disease: In renovascular disease, the arteries supplying blood to the kidneys are affected by Atherosclerosis, potentially compromising kidney function. Like other Atherosclerosis-related conditions, medical management and intervention may be required.

In all these ways that Atherosclerosis can manifest, it's essential to learn about it early and treat it quickly. This helps stop more problems from happening and keeps your organs healthy. The treatment plan usually includes changing your lifestyle, taking medicines, and sometimes even having procedures like putting in a stent or doing a bypass surgery. The main aim is to manage the disease, slow down how quickly it worsens, and improve your life. To do this, it's important to keep visiting the doctor regularly and following their advice. This way, you can manage these blood vessel problems well and lower the chance of having serious issues.

Inflammatory Nonatherosclerotic Vascular Disease (Vasculitis)

Apart from Atherosclerosis, other inflammatory diseases of the blood vessels can lead to serious health issues. Takayasu disease is a rare type of vasculitis that affects the vessels and is characterized by inflammation and narrowing of the arteries. It predominantly affects young female patients and presents with unusual hypertension and blood pressure variations. One arm may experience reduced pulses while the other arm or limbs show incredibly high blood pressure readings. Takayasu disease is a non-atherosclerotic inflammatory condition; the exact cause is unknown. The inflammation causes the vessel endothelium and epithelium to shrink, leading to compromised blood flow. Unlike Atherosclerosis, the inflammation is not related to fat deposits. The characteristic of Takayasu disease involves specific vessels and locations, with the aorta and its branches being more commonly affected, especially in the neck and hands. Due to the slow progression of the disease, patients may not experience symptoms even when the artery is significantly blocked, as collateral circulation may have developed over time. Patients may experience a pulseless condition, indicating a lack of pulse in certain areas. The treatment plan for Takayasu disease is to use medicines. But suppose the problem is terrible, and there's a significant blockage. In that case, the doctors might think about doing a particular procedure like putting in a stent or doing surgery to fix it. Sometimes, if the blockage is long, the stent might not work well, so they might need to do surgery where they take a blood vessel from somewhere else and use it to bypass the blocked area. This disease usually happens in younger people, especially girls. It is crucial for patients with these vascular diseases, whether caused by Atherosclerosis or other inflammatory conditions like Takayasu disease, to adhere to lifelong medical management, lifestyle changes, and regular follow-ups. Proper management and intervention, when needed, can help prevent complications and improve the overall quality of life for those affected.

8

VALVULAR HEART DISEASES

"The strongest hearts have the most scars".

– Jeff Hood

Valvular heart disease is when any valve in the heart has been damaged or is diseased. The valves open and close to provide the unidirectional blood flow from one chamber to the next chamber. They are essential *"transient point"* in blood flow that maintains the serial connection of the left and right heart so that blood collected from the whole body reaches the right atrium, passes to the right ventricle, and then to the pulmonary artery to get purified in the lungs, then reaches the left atrium and finally in left ventricle before ejected into the aorta to supply whole body.

These valves provide one-way traffic to maintain this efficient blood flow. Any compromise in its function will finally lead to heart failure.

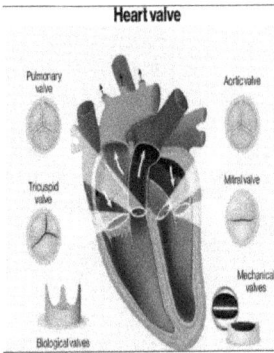

Heart valve

Pulmonary valve
Aortic valve
Tricuspid valve
Mitral valve
Mechanical valves
Biological valves

Valve disease

Valve Stenosis - when the valve opening becomes narrow and restricts blood flow

Valve Prolapse - when a valve slips out of place or the valve flaps (leaflets) does not close properly.

Valve Regurgitation - when blood leaks backwards through a valve, sometimes due to prolapse.

Prosthetic valve

Mechanical valves are made from durable metals, carbon, ceramics and plastics, and patient need lifelong anticoagulant after implant.

Biological valves are made from animal tissue, donated human tissue, or a patient's own tissues. Biological valves are less durable then mechanical valves. Patient doesn't need lifelong anticoagulant

---

Valvular Heart Disease - (Native and Prosthetic Valve)

Valvular heart diseases can be classified into three main categories. The first category comprises congenital valvular heart diseases, present since birth. The second category includes acquired valvular diseases, which can be further divided into two branches: rheumatic heart disease, which occurs in young individuals, and degenerative heart disease, which usually develops in the elderly. These three types of valvular heart diseases are commonly observed in clinical practice.

Congenital Valvular Heart Diseases

When a baby is born with a problem in their heart valve that they got from birth, it's called Congenital valvular disease. Doctors specializing in kids' heart problems can look at specific things to check how the valve works. Sometimes, if the valve is causing trouble with blood flow, the baby might need surgery just a few hours after birth. Before birth, the baby doesn't use its lungs for breathing because the placenta does that job. Everything the baby needs comes from the placenta. But right after birth, the baby's body needs to start using its lungs, so the blood has to flow correctly through the heart. Some heart problems might not appear until after birth because the placenta is still working. However, once the baby is born and disconnected from the placenta, some heart problems can be dangerous and need quick treatment to save the baby's life.

Doctors caring for kids' heart problems are essential in finding and treating these issues. If one baby in a family is born with this kind of problem, there's a higher chance that other babies might have similar or different heart valve problems. Moms need to tell the doctors about any heart problems in their previous pregnancies. This can help the doctors keep an eye on the baby's heart during the current pregnancy, and sometimes, they can even do things to help the baby's heart before it's born.

Luckily, with today's technology, there are different ways to fix these heart problems, like surgery or a particular procedure using a balloon. These treatments can be done on babies who are just born or even while they're still inside their mom's belly. Medicine has advanced so much that doctors can even do treatments while the baby is still in the womb.

Among congenital valvular heart diseases, the aortic and pulmonary valves are the most commonly affected valves, often experiencing complications due to valvular stenosis. Stenosis refers to the abnormal narrowing of a passage. In aortic stenosis, the passage through the aortic valve between the left ventricle and the aorta allows oxygenated blood to flow into the primary artery. Due to stenosis, proper blood flow from the left ventricle into the aorta is hindered. In such situations, balloon surgery or valve replacement may be required. Similar issues can also occur with the mitral valve, which is situated between the left atrium and left ventricle. The treatment options are identical in these cases as well. However, the severity of the disease is carefully assessed by pediatric cardiologists, who consider various parameters, guidelines, and their own experience before deciding on the appropriate course of action.

Each case is unique, and factors like patient symptoms, age, weight, valve severity, and chamber morphology are considered before determining whether immediate intervention is necessary or if the condition can be managed more cautiously. A collaborative decision-making process involving a team of pediatric doctors, pediatric cardiologists, and pediatric surgeons is followed, especially for newborn babies, to ensure the best possible treatment plan is implemented.

Rheumatic Valvular Heart Diseases

The second type of valvular heart disease, more common in developing countries than developed ones, is an acquired heart disease called rheumatic heart disease. This condition typically develops young, usually between 5 and 15 years. The underlying cause of rheumatic heart disease is an infection known as acute rheumatic fever. Following this infection, children or teenagers may experience symptoms such as migratory multiple-joint pain (moving from one joint to another in 1-2 weeks). It is preceded by cough or cold-like symptoms and fever, which may not be severe enough and go unnoticed. However, in most cases, the valve abnormality gets noticed after years or decades of initial acute illness, in which those mentioned above, typical joint pain is the only way to pinpoint the initial insult of this disease. The heart valve's inflammatory response sets in that period and is a gradually progressive disorder more like a smoldering inflammation of the valve, which manifests later on as valve stenosis or regurgitation. Stenosis refers to a narrowing of the valve, while regurgitation means leaking. Occasionally, both conditions can co-occur in single or multiple valves, which is incredibly unique to this disease.

Rheumatic fever can affect the valves in the heart, and the most common one it affects is called the mitral valve. This can cause problems like the valve getting narrow (mitral stenosis), the valve leaking (mitral regurgitation), or both things happening together. Other valves, like the aortic and tricuspid valves, can also be affected, but it's not as common, and the pulmonary valve is rarely involved.

One sign of mitral stenosis is feeling short of breath when you're active; we use the term dyspnoea on exertion(DOE). People with rheumatic fever when they are 5 to 15 years old might start feeling this way in their 20s after many years. Doctors can often determine if someone has a valve problem by examining their medical history and doing tests like an ECG and echocardiography. An experienced doctor can see the kind of valve problem, specifically related to rheumatic disease, using an echocardiogram. Echocardiography is enough to make the diagnosis, so extra blood tests aren't usually needed. For both kids and adults, echocardiography is the primary test to check for valve problems in the heart. It helps doctors see all four valves and how serious the problem is, which is essential for deciding the best treatment. This could be a less invasive procedure called valvuloplasty (minimally invasive balloon surgery) or a more extensive surgery where they replace the valve.

Echocardiography is a gold standard test to establish or rule out if someone has a valve problem, like how angiography is the best way to check for problems in the arteries. While an ECG can give some hints, echocardiography provides a clear and complete picture of what's going on, which helps doctors make good treatment decisions.

Rheumatic valve disease usually gets worse slowly after someone has rheumatic fever as a kid. The most common thing that happens is the mitral valve gets narrow, which makes it hard to breathe when you're active. Sometimes, this narrow valve can make the right side of the heart work too hard, and that can cause other problems like the tricuspid valve leaking. This can lead to feeling full in the belly and having swollen feet. If a young person has trouble breathing and swollen feet, it could be because of a problem with the left side of their heart (either a valve or muscle problem), causing the right side of the heart not to work well. In pediatric and adult cases, echocardiography is the primary diagnostic tool for valvular heart disease. It allows visualization of all four valves of the heart and the severity of each valve abnormality, which is crucial in finalizing the management path.

Based on this information, treatment options can be determined, such as minimally invasive valvoplasty (also called balloon valve surgery) and valve replacement, which requires a surgeon or medical management to do open heart surgery.

Echocardiography is the gold standard for diagnosing valvular heart disease, just as angiography is for coronary artery disease. While ECG can provide some clues, echocardiography offers a comprehensive and definitive picture of the condition, allowing for precise and effective management decisions.

Rheumatic valvular disease progresses slowly after an episode of rheumatic fever in childhood, and the most common manifestation is mitral stenosis, leading to breathlessness on exertion. Additionally, mitral stenosis can cause a back pressure effect on the right side of the heart, resulting in tricuspid regurgitation. This can lead to symptoms such as fullness in the abdomen and pedal edema or swelling in the feet. The combination of breathlessness and swelling in the feet in a young patient often indicates left heart disease (either valve or muscle disease), leading to right heart failure until proven otherwise.

In cases of predominantly aortic stenosis, patients may experience three key complaints: breathlessness, giddiness, and syncope (fainting attacks). If a young patient without any risk factors for coronary artery disease experiences chest pain and breathlessness, the possibility of heart disease, specifically aortic stenosis, is significantly higher. Long-term symptoms of chest pain, breathlessness, and syncope in aortic stenosis can indicate the development of heart failure, which can sometimes be fatal. However, if not severe, some patients with aortic stenosis may not experience any symptoms, necessitating careful clinical evaluation and echocardiogram correlation.

In the case of rheumatic heart disease, it is possible for back pressure to affect the right side of the heart whenever the left side is involved. This can lead to features such as swelling of the feet and easy fatigability. Additionally, enlargement of the liver may cause abdominal fullness and swelling too. The progression of rheumatic heart disease is typically slower, with symptoms starting to manifest between 18 and 20 years of age and progressing over the next one or two decades.

A multidisciplinary team of medical professionals considers the patient's symptoms, echocardiographic findings, and severity of valve dysfunction to determine the appropriate course of action for valve disease. Timely intervention through surgical or percutaneous procedures can significantly improve the patient's prognosis and quality of life.

Echocardiography plays a critical role in diagnosing and assessing the severity of valvular heart diseases. In severe cases of stenosis or regurgitation, a valve replacement may be necessary, particularly if the patient is experiencing symptoms.

Treatment of Rheumatic Valve Disease

Mild to moderate valve disease - Medical management is the primary approach for mild to moderate valve disease, whether mitral or aortic, stenotic or regurgitation of the valve. Medications are used to modify the condition and relieve the symptoms. A three-weekly Penidure injection containing Benzathine penicillin is a very effective treatment in reducing the progression of valve dysfunction by reducing the likelihood of recurrent rheumatic fever attacks. It has to be continued till the age of 45. Preventing further attacks is essential, as each episode can exacerbate valve stenosis or regurgitation.

Severe Valve disease

Mitral valve disease – For *mitral stenosis*, balloon surgery, in which a balloon is percutaneously used to open the valve, may be an option if the valve area is significantly reduced (defined as valve area <1cm2). However, in cases of severe *mitral regurgitation* and any rise in pulmonary arterial pressure or development of atrial fibrillation, it marks a turning point in mitral valve disease. Hence, a valve replacement is often required and should be planned early.

Aortic valve disease - Aortic regurgitation is another critical condition where the valve fails to prevent blood from flowing back into the left ventricle instead of propelling it into the aorta. Like mitral valve disease, aortic stenosis, and aortic regurgitation, aortic regurgitation also requires valve replacement. When a patient presents with symptoms of valve disease along with severe valve dysfunction (mitral and aortic) defined by echocardiogram criteria in the guideline, then they are a candidate for a native valve replacement with mechanical or bioprosthetic valve except for mitral stenosis where balloon surgery is still an option if the valve morphology is suitable.

Rheumatic heart disease is caused by specific streptococcus strain infection, and recurrent infections can lead to valve damage over time. Thus, ongoing prevention and management of infectious attacks are critical to mitigating disease progression and preserving valve function.

Typically occurring between the ages of 15 and 50, rheumatic heart disease requires careful monitoring and long-term management to improve patient outcomes and quality of life.

Degenerative Valvular Heart Diseases

Degenerative heart disease, the third type of valvular heart disease, usually develops at an older age, typically in the 60s or later. These conditions arise from the natural aging process, as the valves degenerate and accumulate calcium and fibrosis. The progression of degenerative heart disease varies from person to person and is influenced by genetics and other risk factors like diabetes, hypertension, and smoking. Research is ongoing to understand why some individuals may develop these conditions earlier in life while others experience them much later.

Among degenerative heart diseases, the aortic valve is most commonly affected. The aortic valve between the aorta and the left ventricle thickens and develops calcium deposits, leading to compromised blood flow and increased pressure gradient. Traditionally, open heart valve replacement surgery with bypass support was the only available treatment option for aortic stenosis for a considerable period.

However, advancements in medical technology have introduced a less invasive alternative known as Transcatheter Aortic Valve Replacement (TAVR). This procedure inserts a percutaneous valve directly into the stenosed area through the aorta without open heart surgery. This percutaneous valve replaces the compromised valve and restores normal blood flow. TAVR is especially preferred for high-risk patients for conventional surgery due to anesthesia-related risks or other comorbidities. TAVR offers a viable option for these individuals with a shorter hospital stay, often just one day.

While TAVR is a remarkable advancement in treating aortic stenosis, it is still primarily recommended for patients who cannot undergo conventional surgery. As research and technology progress, TAVR may become a more widely used and accessible option for all patients with aortic stenosis.

Valvular heart diseases are specific problems with the valves in the heart, and they can show up at different times in life. One of these diseases involves the bicuspid aortic valve, which some people are born with. Usually, the aortic valve has three leaflets, but only two are in these cases. As time goes on, this valve might start leaking or getting narrower. When it mostly starts leaking before the age of 50, it is called aortic regurgitation, and when it narrows, which happens in patients older than 60, it is called aortic stenosis. Sometimes, leakiness and narrowing can occur along with a problem in the aorta. These patients can develop aortic dissection (tear in aorta) or aortic aneurysm (blowing out of aorta), the significant blood vessel connected to the heart. This can make the aorta bigger and cause bleeding inside, which is terrible for the body's circulation. It's interesting because this disease is something you're born with, but it might not cause any issues until later in life.

Doctors usually use an echocardiography test to determine if someone has a problem with their heart valves. This helps them see what's going on with the valves. There are three types of valve problems: ones you're born with, ones that come from infections when you're young, and ones that develop as you age.

These problems mainly affect two valves on the left side of the heart, the mitral and aortic valves. If the mitral valve gets narrow, it can make breathing difficult and manifest as a breathing problem. If it leaks, it can cause trouble breathing, fast heartbeats, and heart failure. If the aortic valve narrows, you might feel heavy in your chest, have trouble breathing, and even get dizzy. If it leaks, you might feel your heart racing, especially when lying down.

Echocardiography is essential to determine if someone has a valve problem. If they do, the doctors can figure out the best way to help, like fixing or replacing the valve. This can make life better for people with these heart issues. Right-sided heart diseases typically don't present many symptoms and are often associated with left-sided heart diseases. However, in rare cases, we encounter conditions that solely affect the right side of the heart without involving the left side. The common complaints in such cases are valve leaking, lower limb swelling, and easy fatigability.

The pulmonary valve in the right ventricle is least likely to be affected by diseases other than congenital conditions. Symptoms for isolated pulmonary valve diseases, such as pulmonary stenosis or regurgitation, may include breathlessness. Echocardiography is crucial for confirming any isolated pulmonary valve disease, as it is mostly seen in pediatric cases and rarely in survived adults.

When a valve is affected by infection or disease, it can also impact the related heart chambers, leading to chamber dilation. A leaky or narrowed valve creates pressure on the chamber walls, weakening the muscles. The chamber upstream to the affected valve will dilate due to increased pressure. For instance, in mitral stenosis, where the mitral valve is narrowed, there will be high pressure on the left atrium, causing dilation. This, in turn, leads to breathlessness, as the left atrium collects oxygenated blood from the lungs, and the blocked mitral valve exerts back pressure on the lungs. In mitral regurgitation, where the valve is leaky, the left atrium and left ventricle may dilate, causing low-pressure symptoms, such as easy fatigability.

Surgical valve replacement is the ultimate treatment for severe valve defects. Worldwide accepted criteria, guided by echocardiogram, help determine whether a valve defect is mild, moderate, or severe. Suppose a particular valve defect is associated with severe symptoms like breathlessness, easy fatigability, palpitations, or angina. In that case, that valve can be replaced using open heart surgical procedures or, in specific cases, the less invasive Transcatheter Aortic Valve Replacement (TAVR) procedure, especially for older patients.

9

HEART MUSCLE DISEASES
(CARDIOMYOPATHY)

"Heart failure may weaken the heart muscle, but it can never weaken the
determination to live and thrive."

- Unknown

The heart is composed of a specialized muscle called the myocardium, which plays a vital role in heart function. Its primary function is to facilitate the contraction and relaxation of the heart walls and chambers, enabling the heart to receive and pump blood to all bodily organs. The myocardial cells have distinctive features. The lower chambers(ventricle), which share a common wall (interventricular septum), contract synchronously to generate the ideal force to pump blood in the systemic and pulmonary circulation. This contraction (*systole*) is followed by proper relaxation(*diastole*), ensuring efficient blood circulation throughout the body. Therefore, any diseases affecting the myocardium can be highly critical and even life-threatening.

Cardiomyopathies, variants of myocardial heart disease, can broadly be categorized into Hypertrophic Cardiomyopathy and

Dilated Cardiomyopathy. Similarly, impairment of systolic function leads to Heart failure with reduced ejection fraction (HFrEF), while impairment of proper diastolic filling leads to heart failure with preserved ejection fraction (HFpEF). There is a condition called restrictive cardiomyopathy, where the diastolic filling is compromised due to infiltration or fibrosis in cardiac muscle. To avoid confusion, we are restricting to the most common myocardial diseases.

Hypertrophic Cardiomyopathy (HCM)

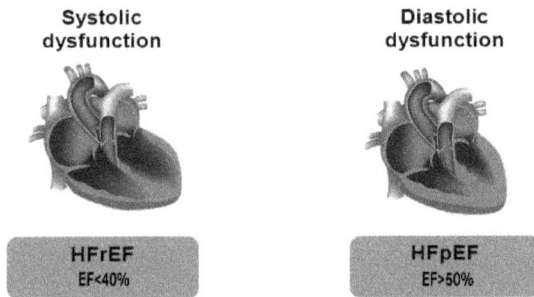

Systolic dysfunction

Diastolic dysfunction

HFrEF EF<40%

HFpEF EF>50%

Types of Heart Failure

The thickening of the heart muscle characterizes hypertrophic cardiomyopathy (HCM) (increase in muscle mass without any cause), making it challenging for the heart to pump blood effectively. It is often asymptomatic and can go undiagnosed due to its subtle nature. HCM is primarily attributed to genetic factors, which develop later in life due to inherited genes within the family. Studies suggest that approximately one out of every 500 individuals may have HCM, making it one of the most common heart diseases.

In patients with HCM, their heart appears normal during childhood and adolescence. However, over time, the heart muscle hypertrophy or thickens disproportionately without any specific cause. It is essential to differentiate HCM from congenital heart diseases, abnormalities present from birth. HCM is linked explicitly to genetic factors and not congenital conditions.

While hypertrophy can also occur in individuals with hypertension or valve diseases like aortic valve disease, HCM occurs in patients without these conditions. In this disease, the heart muscle multiplies and thickens, leading to compromised heart function. Hypertrophy can affect the heart chambers and adversely affect mitral valve function, reducing their capacity to hold blood (*diastolic filling*) and causing obstruction in the smooth flow through the valves and mitral valve leak (mitral regurgitation).

A significant concern in HCM is the development of a dynamic obstruction just below the aortic valve, known as Left Ventricular Outflow Tract Obstruction (LVOTO). During the heart's contraction, the blood flow through the aortic valve is hindered by the squeeze of the chamber muscle beneath the valve. This dynamic obstruction compromises blood flow to the aorta, leading to circulation issues. Over time, LVOTO can also cause changes in the mitral valve leaflet apparatus, resulting in regurgitation or leakage of blood. Early detection and management of HCM are crucial to preventing complications and ensuring proper heart function. Echocardiography plays a vital role in diagnosing this condition and evaluating its severity.

In hypertrophic cardiomyopathy (HCM), the thickening of the heart muscle can lead to symptoms resembling aortic stenosis and mitral regurgitation. The dynamic obstruction below the aortic valve, called Left Ventricular Outflow Tract Obstruction (LVOTO), causes difficulty for blood to be pushed into the aorta. Additionally, the hypertrophy can result in mitral valve regurgitation, further complicating the heart's function. The combination of these conditions typically presents with three significant symptoms: angina (chest pain), breathlessness, and syncope (fainting). In severe cases, sudden death can also be a possibility.

When the heart muscle becomes thicker (a condition called hypertrophy), it might not get enough blood because the arteries can't reach all the thickened parts. This lack of blood can cause scars in the heart muscle, which can then cause serious rhythm problems like Ventricular Tachycardia (VT) or Ventricular Fibrillation (VF). These rhythm problems make the heart's electrical signals go haywire and can lead to the heart suddenly stopping, called cardiac arrest. This can happen suddenly, especially in young people. It's a big reason why some athletes and non-athletes can suddenly collapse and die, even if they seem healthy. HCM is a genetic disease that can run in families. Valuable information can be gained by studying the family pedigree. If there has been a history of sudden death in a first-degree relative, it alerts healthcare providers to examine family members for potential symptoms carefully. Early detection and management are vital in HCM to prevent complications and provide appropriate treatment and monitoring for affected individuals and their family members.

Hypertrophic cardiomyopathy (HCM) is a common genetic disease that runs in families, and it can be unpredictable and life-threatening due to the risk of sudden cardiac arrest. While initially, medical management is attempted based on the severity of the disease, patients with a history of cardiac arrest, VT, and VF are considered ideal candidates for an Implantable Cardioverter Defibrillator (ICD) implantation. The ICD is a life-saving device that can revive the patient, particularly those with an episode of cardiac arrest, VT/ VF, syncope, and a family history of SCD, as it can detect life-threatening rhythm disorder and aborts cardiac arrest in case of future arrhythmias.

Medical management for HCM typically involves prescribing beta-blockers and other drugs like disopyramide (Norpace) to reduce muscle contraction and alleviate compromised circulation. However, in cases where symptoms persist despite medication, surgical interventions are considered. Transaortic Septal Myectomy is a surgical procedure in which the surgeon removes hypertrophic muscle mass from the left ventricle to improve circulation and alleviate symptoms. Percutaneous alcohol ablation is a less invasive procedure where alcohol is introduced into a specific region of the heart muscle to create controlled myocardial infarction, reducing hypertrophy and improving dynamic obstruction.

Diagnosing HCM is relatively straightforward. An electrocardiogram (ECG) often shows classical features of the disease in around 90% of cases. However, an echocardiogram (Echo) is the primary diagnostic tool to confirm or rule out heart muscle or valve diseases. In some cases where the diagnosis is unclear or the patient has no symptoms, a Cardiac MRI may be required for a more comprehensive evaluation of the heart's muscles and contraction patterns.

HCM is a genetic disease with potentially severe consequences. Still, early detection and appropriate management, including ICD implantation and surgical interventions, can significantly improve the patient's outlook and quality of life. Due to their hereditary nature, regular monitoring and follow-up with healthcare professionals are essential for those with HCM and their family members.

Dilated Cardiomyopathy (DCM)

Dilated Cardiomyopathy (DCM) is the opposite of Hypertrophic Cardiomyopathy (HCM). In DCM, the heart muscles become thinner and dilated (expand in dimension) without a clear cause. Some studies suggest that it might be related to a past viral illness that triggered inflammation in the heart, leading to progressive weakening of the heart muscle and dilation of its chambers, especially the left ventricle. As the heart muscle weakens and becomes thin, the chamber size increases, leading to reduced pumping pressure and compromised circulation.

As the disease progresses, the dilated chambers can affect the function of the heart valves, causing them to expand and separate, resulting in mitral valve regurgitation (leakage). Additionally, DCM can be associated with an electrical problem called Left Bundle Branch Block (LBBB), which further contributes to compromised heart function.

The presentation of DCM is characterized by gradually increasing breathlessness. Patients may initially experience mild symptoms during exertion, but the level of breathlessness worsens over time. Eventually, patients may develop Paroxysmal Nocturnal Dyspnea (PND), where they wake up after a few hours of sleep gasping for breath and may have to sit up to find relief. This condition can severely disrupt sleep, making it difficult for patients to lie comfortably in the supine position.

If DCM goes untreated, it can also progress to involve the right side of the heart. This can lead to pedal edema, where the feet swell, reduced appetite, and decreased urination. These features collectively indicate the development of advanced heart failure.

Diagnosing DCM is primarily done through echocardiography (Echo), which allows visualization of the heart's structure and function. Treatment for DCM aims to manage symptoms, slow down disease progression, and improve heart function. Medications, such as angiotensin-converting enzyme (ACE) inhibitors, beta-blockers, and diuretics, are commonly prescribed to improve heart function, control blood pressure, and reduce fluid retention.

In some cases, advanced heart failure due to DCM may require more aggressive interventions, such as implantable devices like a biventricular pacemaker or cardiac resynchronization therapy (CRT), to optimize heart function and improve symptoms. In severe cases, heart transplantation may be considered as a last resort.

Regular monitoring and follow-up with a healthcare professional are essential for patients with DCM to manage the disease effectively and optimize their quality of life.

Dilated Cardiomyopathy (DCM) represents the final stage of heart failure, known as Heart Failure with reduced Ejection Fraction (HFrEF). Ejection fraction indicates the percentage of blood ejected from a chamber during a single contraction. In DCM, the heart's left ventricle becomes enlarged, and the mitral valve may also become leaky. The severity of heart failure is assessed based on the left ventricular ejection fraction. An ejection fraction of 55% to 60% is considered normal, while values between 45% to 55%, 35% to 45%, and less than 35% are classified as mild, moderate, and severe heart failure, respectively. However, a new classification has emerged, dividing the ejection fraction range into 40% to 50% for Heart Failure with preserved Ejection Fraction (HFpEF) and less than 40% for HFrEF.

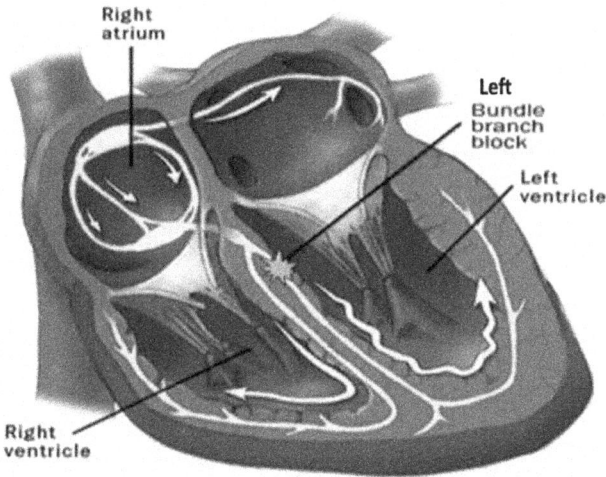

The treatment approach for DCM involves utilizing four primary drugs: ACE (Angiotensin-converting Enzyme) inhibitors/ARNI(Angiotensin receptor blocker with Naprilysin inhibitor), MRAs (Mineralocorticoid Receptor Antagonists), beta-blockers, and SGLT2 (Sodium-glucose Cotransporter-2) inhibitors. These drugs are combined with diuretics to reduce salt and water retention. Digtoxin is also prescribed to assist the heart in normal contraction. Early intervention with these medications can help prevent further heart damage. In case of infections or other complications, prompt treatment is essential to minimize risks during any surgical intervention.

Additional options are available for patients who do not respond to medications. Patients with heart failure and having left bundle branch block (LBBB) on their ECG may undergo Cardiac Resynchronization Therapy (CRT) device implantation. Those

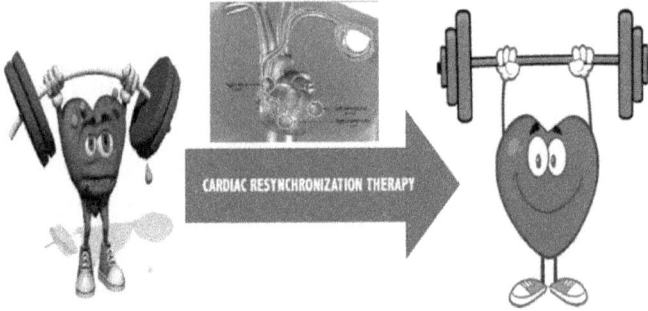

without LBBB may receive a Left Ventricular Assist Device (LVAD), which assists the left ventricle's contraction to maintain blood circulation. The LVAD can act as a bridge therapy for patients awaiting heart transplantation. Heart transplantation is considered the ultimate treatment option for suitable candidates under 60 or 65 with healthy other organ functions. After a successful transplant, patients can enjoy a longevity of 15 to 25 years, depending on individual circumstances and lifestyle choices.

In conclusion, Dilated Cardiomyopathy represents the end stage of heart failure, and patients may require progressive treatments depending on their response to medications and specific cardiac conditions. CRT or LVAD implantation may be appropriate for some, while others may ultimately undergo heart transplantation. DCM can arise from various underlying causes, including valvular, electrical, and ischemic heart diseases. Nevertheless, with early detection and appropriate management, the progression of DCM can be delayed, improving patients' overall prognosis.

Heart transplantation is the last treatment option when someone's heart is weak and not working well. This happens when the heart is failing and can't pump blood effectively. There are two types of this condition: one where the heart pumps even weaker (called "reduced ejection fraction") and another where the pumping is not too weak but still can't handle enough blood ("preserved ejection fraction"). To treat this, doctors use different methods, like giving medicines, using a special device called left ventricular Assisted device (LVAD) to help the heart, or even doing a heart transplant, which means replacing the weak heart with a healthier one. The heart's pumping is less weak in heart failure with preserved ejection fraction. However, it still fails to accommodate and process the required amount of blood, leading to symptoms like breathlessness on exertion and pedal edema. Treatments for heart failure with preserved ejection fraction are medications and aggressive comorbidity correction. We have no good medication for HFpEF except SGLT2i, which was recently approved for this disease. It is primarily an effect of uncontrolled morbidities (diabetes, hypertension, COPD, obesity, CKD, etc.), which adversely affect the heart's diastolic filling function. Hence, correction of uncontrolled comorbidity is sheet anchor treatment of this type of heart failure (HFpEF).

Heart Transplant

Transplantation is the ultimate treatment for advanced heart failure, categorized into four stages from A to D.

1. Stage A represents the early stage with risk factors such as diabetes or hypertension but no heart failure symptoms.
2. Stage B indicates the presence of risk factors and mild heart failure, still allowing the patient to carry out daily activities without significant difficulty.
3. In Stage C, the heart is dilated and exhibits heart failure symptoms but responds to medical treatment.
4. Lastly, Stage D, known as refractory heart failure, signifies compromised heart chambers and unresponsiveness to medications.

Patients in stages C and D are typically considered candidates for a heart transplant. A heart transplant can significantly prolong their life when medical and device management prove ineffective, and other organs function well. However, extensive tests are performed before the transplant procedure to ensure the patient's suitability for the surgery. Additionally, the condition of the lungs is assessed, as they are situated near the heart.

The donor heart is typically obtained from a brain-dead individual and must be transplanted within a few hours. The heart transplantation process is complex and requires collaboration among cardiologists, electrophysiologists, and cardiothoracic surgeons. Following the transplant surgery, the patient is prescribed immunosuppressant medications for a certain period, and any signs of acute or chronic rejections are closely monitored. Usually, within three to six months, the new heart becomes fully integrated into the recipient's body.

Arrhythmogenic Right Ventricular Dysplasia (ARVD)

While we have primarily discussed left-sided cardiomyopathies, some conditions affect the right side of the heart. One such condition is Arrhythmogenic Right Ventricular Dysplasia (ARVD), a rare but potentially lethal disease.

In ARVD, fatty tissue in the right ventricle gradually replaces the heart tissue, compromising the heart's ability to pump blood efficiently. This fatty infiltration weakens the heart muscle and can lead to dangerous arrhythmias, such as ventricular tachycardia (VT) and ventricular fibrillation (VF), which can cause sudden cardiac arrest. ARVD is known to be a significant cause of sudden death in young athletes, and early diagnosis is crucial for timely management and intervention.

The exact cause of ARVD is not fully understood, but it is a genetic disease that sometimes runs in the family. In this disease, fatty infiltration happens in the right ventricle, which weakens the right ventricle and leads to electrical abnormalities and potentially fatal arrhythmias.

Despite its potential severity, ARVD remains under-recognized and often misdiagnosed. The symptoms of ARVD can be subtle and easily mistaken for other heart conditions. However, a careful evaluation of the patient's medical history and family history and thorough cardiac tests, including electrocardiogram (ECG) and echocardiogram, can aid in identifying the disease.

Treatment for ARVD is multifaceted and depends on the disease's phase and severity. Like other cardiomyopathies, the first line of treatment involves medications, such as beta-blockers and anti-arrhythmic drugs, to manage symptoms and prevent arrhythmias. Additionally, implantable devices like the Automatic Implantable Cardioverter Defibrillator (AICD) can detect and correct life-threatening arrhythmias. The AICD safeguards against sudden cardiac arrest, providing immediate electrical shocks when necessary to restore normal heart rhythm.

For some patients with advanced ARVD, heart transplantation may be the final option. Heart transplantation is complex, and candidates must meet specific eligibility criteria. Younger patients with well-functioning other organs, such as lungs and kidneys, are more likely to be considered for heart transplantation.

Diagnosing cardiomyopathies can be challenging, as the symptoms may overlap with other heart conditions. However, modern diagnostic tools and advances in medical technology, such as cardiac MRI, have greatly improved the accuracy of diagnosis. For instance, cardiac MRI can reveal structural and functional changes in the heart muscle that may not be apparent in routine echocardiograms.

Genetic testing also plays a crucial role in diagnosing specific cardiomyopathies, including hypertrophic cardiomyopathy and ARVD. Identifying specific genetic mutations can provide valuable insights into the disease's progression, prognosis, and risk of complications.

In summary, cardiomyopathies are a diverse group of heart muscle diseases affecting the heart's left and right sides. Early and accurate diagnosis is essential for appropriate treatment and preventing life-threatening complications. Advances in medical technology and genetic testing have revolutionized the diagnosis and management of these conditions, allowing for personalized and targeted therapies. Cardiomyopathies may present complex challenges, but with a comprehensive and multidisciplinary approach, patients can achieve improved outcomes and a better quality of life.

One of my patients is a 36-year-old woman who used to have recurring near-death experiences while playing with her child. She used to feel giddiness while chasing after her child. But then, out of nowhere, it became so bad that she lost consciousness for a few moments and was not breathing during this time. It's like her body hits pause, and then, miraculously, she returns to life.

Here's the eerie part: she can't remember what happened during those blackout moments. All she could describe was a wild sensation of her heart pounding, followed by everything swirling around her. It's like she's caught in a tremendous amount of confusion. But this isn't the first time it's happened; it's struck her twice before, with a four-month gap between episodes. It was a recurring nightmare. Thanks to an ECHO test, a closer look revealed a condition known as ARVD (Arrhythmogenic Right Ventricular Dysplasia). Her heart has some issues with its rhythm, and it can sometimes go haywire, especially when she's physically active. Here's where it gets imperative: when she has these episodes and her heart stops, then magically starts again on its own, we call it a cardiac arrest with spontaneous recovery. Overall, it is a scary experience.

But, if things get even more serious, and she would need CPR or a shock to get her heart back in the game. It's a reminder that the heart's rhythm can sometimes go off track, and it's good that we (doctors and medical professionals) are around to bring it back to life.

10

ARRHYTHMIAS OR RHYTHM DISORDERS

"You will never be able to escape from your heart. So it's better to listen to what it has to say. That way, you'll never have to fear an unanticipated blow."

-Paulo Coelho (The Alchemist)

As discussed earlier, the heart's function relies on its rhythmic beating, which is produced by its electrical system. In simpler terms, we refer to this as the heartbeat. This harmonious rhythm, in conjunction with respiration, ensures that oxygen-rich blood is promptly distributed to all body systems, making the heart's rhythm crucial for our overall health.

Heartbeat- The regular movement of the heart by which it pumps the blood around our body is called a heartbeat. It is the defining feature of the beginning of personal human life. The cardiovascular system is the *first organ system* to function, and the human embryonic heart starts beating 22 days after fertilization, corresponding to 36th days of gestation(7th week of pregnancy). These contractions appear as small, irregular twitches within circumscribed areas of the developing myocardium and do not generate coordinated movements of the developing heart that cause fluid flow.

From all the organs of our body, the heart and the brain have received an eminent position in the diverse philosophical, theological, and biomedical concepts of human life. Each of the two organs was proposed as the soul's location or the source of the "vital principle" that defined personal human life. The heart or the brain as the source of the vital principle significantly impacts the practical work in medical terminology. This is because the presence of heart or brain activity can be regarded as an indicator of life. The irreversible cessation of heart or brain activity can then be viewed as the defining sign of the death of an individual human being. Till the 1960s, the traditional legal definition of death in most parts of the world was the cessation of cardio-respiratory function. During the late 1960s, the medicolegal definition of death shifted from a heart-centered to a brain-centered definition of death, significantly impacting the development of transplantation medicine. The IPC(Indian Panel Code)-46 defines death in the Indian constitution, and its Section 2(e) defines the Transplantation of Human Organs Act (THOA, 1994) — Death is 'the permanent disappearance of all evidence of life because of brainstem death or in a cardiopulmonary sense at any time after live birth has taken.

Arrhythmia

Arrhythmia, also known as a rhythm disorder, occurs when there is an abnormality in the heart's beating caused by an electrical problem. It can manifest as a primary disease, where the rhythm disorder is the primary disorder and is not the manifestation of another heart disease. Alternatively, it can be a secondary phenomenon resulting from valve, muscle, or coronary disease.

Dizziness	Sudden cardiac death
Palpitation	
Fainting	Paroxysmal sweating with weakness

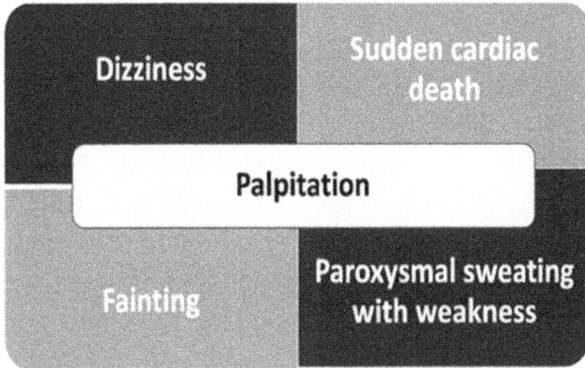

Symptoms of Arrhythmia (Electrical Problem) or Heartbeat Problems

Before delving into specific types of arrhythmias, let's revisit the normal process of current generation and conduction through the heart muscle that facilitates its rhythmic contraction and relaxation. Remarkably, a forming heart begins its first beating on the 22nd day post-fertilization inside a mother's womb when a child is conceived. The Sinoatrial node (SA node) is pivotal in generating the electrical stimulus for initiating the heartbeat. It is located in the right atrium and possesses the intrinsic ability to produce this electrical impulse throughout life without fail.

With arrhythmias, the primary symptom is palpitation, but it can also manifest as giddiness, syncope, or fainting attacks. In some cases, an unexplained fracture or injury in elderly patients may be linked to tachyarrhythmia, causing sudden fainting and subsequent falls leading to injuries. Often, arrhythmic evaluation is overlooked in these situations, resulting in missed diagnosis and potentially cardiac arrest or death later on. Hence, any unprovoked injury or head injury, regardless of age, warrants investigation by an electrophysiologist to prevent the risk of sudden death.

Arrhythmias can also affect infants, presenting as seizure disorders or fits. In such cases, treating the symptoms with medication for fits is ineffective, as the problem lies in the heart's rhythm, compromising circulation to the brain. Correctly diagnosing the underlying arrhythmia is crucial for providing appropriate treatment and improving the baby's condition.

Let's discuss a unique and puzzling scenario of this disease I treated. A 12-year-old girl came to see us because she kept fainting while playing, but the real head-scratcher was that she would bounce back on her own. This had been going on since she was a little kid. It seemed like these episodes usually occurred when she pushed herself too hard, going beyond her limits. She gave us the lowdown on her history, which was crucial.

So, we decided to run some tests, including a TMT (Treadmill Test). During this test, something unusual happened – her heart decided to throw a little tantrum, called polymorphic VT (a fancy term for a specific type of irregular heartbeat). This led us to a diagnosis of CPVT, which is short for a mouthful: Catecholaminergic Polymorphic Ventricular Tachycardia. Now, don't let the name scare you because there is good news for this girl. We gave her the correct set of medicines, and those fainting episodes have become a thing of the past. Her heart is back in the game, and she's playing like a champ without any worrisome attacks in sight!

In summary, medications are typically the first-line treatment for various rhythm disorders. Curative treatments such as EP study RF ablation and cryoablation are considered for specific arrhythmias. At the same time, device therapy, like AICD or CRTD, is used in cases of structural heart disease with ventricular tachyarrhythmias and cardiac arrest. It is essential to tailor the treatment plan based on the individual's condition and type of arrhythmia for the best possible outcome.

From the SA node, the current flows through specific channels to reach the Atrioventricular node (AV node), which acts as a transmitter of the heart, regulating the electrical signals from the upper chamber(atrium) to the lower chamber(ventricle).

AV node function*s as a safety valve* in the conduction system. It prevents atrial fibrillation from becoming ventricular fibrillation (killer rhythm) by preventing the very high heart rate of the upper chamber during atrial fibrillation from flowing through it to the lower chamber. The AV node is connected to the lower chamber via bundle His and divided into two major branches. These bundle branches supply electricity to the muscles of the right and left ventricles, allowing them to contract effectively. The heart's normal functioning of this electrical circuit (SA node, AV node, His bundle, Right bundle branch, and left bundle branch) is essential for maintaining a normal heart rhythm. Any compromise in either the electricity generation at the SA node or the conduction at the AV node or bundle branches can lead to a serious heart problem.

Arrhythmias can manifest in various ways, including tachycardia (fast heartbeat), bradycardia (slow heartbeat), atrial fibrillation (irregular and rapid heartbeat), and ventricular fibrillation (chaotic and ineffective heartbeat). These abnormal rhythms can significantly impact the heart's ability to pump blood effectively, leading to symptoms like palpitations, dizziness, fainting, shortness of breath, and, in severe cases, sudden cardiac arrest.

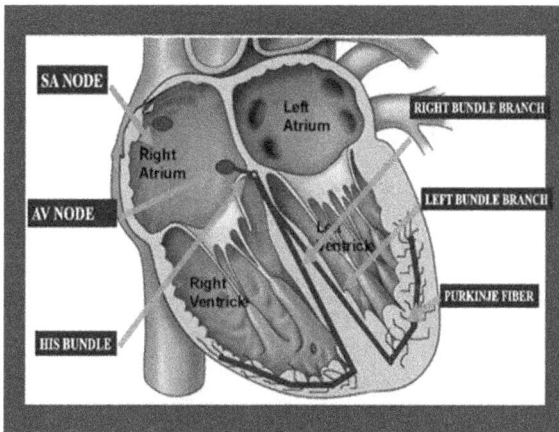

Cardiac Electrical Circuit (Current flow from Generator to Transmitter)

To diagnose arrhythmias, various tests and non-invasive methods such as electrocardiograms (ECGs), Holter monitoring, event monitors, and invasive electrophysiology studies are used to assess the heart's electrical activity. Different treatment options may be recommended based on the specific type and severity of the arrhythmia.

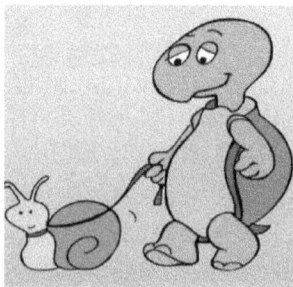

Treatment for arrhythmias can include medications to regulate heart rhythm, procedures like catheter ablation to target and eliminate abnormal electrical circuits, and, in some cases, the implantation of devices like pacemakers or implantable cardioverter-defibrillators (ICDs) to maintain normal heart rhythms or provide immediate correction in case of dangerous arrhythmias.

In summary, the heart's rhythm, driven by its intrinsic electrical system, is vital for maintaining proper cardiac function and overall health. Arrhythmias, or rhythm disorders, can arise from various causes and significantly affect the heart's ability to pump blood effectively. Proper diagnosis and appropriate management of arrhythmias are essential to prevent complications and ensure the well-being of patients with these conditions.

Bradyarrhythmia   **Tachyarrhythmia**

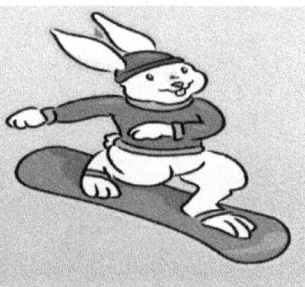

Two categories of rhythm disorders manifest directly without any other primary heart diseases. One is Bradyarrhythmia, and the other is Tachyarrhythmia. Bradyarrhythmia is characterized by a slow heart rhythm or beating rate, while a high heart rate defines tachyarrhythmia.

Brady Arrhythmia

Bradyarrhythmia can occur in two ways. The first is when the electrical current is not formed correctly, leading to reduced electricity generation at the SA node, which is the heart's natural pacemaker. This condition is more commonly observed in older individuals, typically those above 65. As the heart rate gradually decreases, from around a resting heart rate of 140 /min in neonates to adults of 60 to 80/min, it can drop to 50 to 60/min in very elderly persons. If the heart rate drops to a lower rate or the heart's rate behavior becomes unpredictable, it is called sick sinus syndrome. It may start beating very fast and then suddenly slow down. These two phases of the same disease are known as Sick Sinus Syndrome, with both Tachy and Brady rhythms.

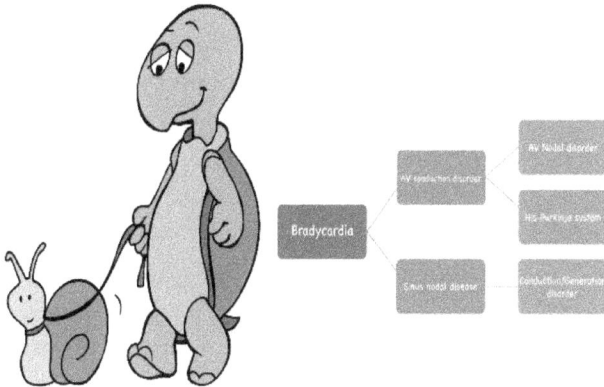

Causes of Bradyarrhythmia (slow heart beating)

Sick Sinus Syndrome presents with complaints of dizziness, palpitations, and fainting attacks. Sometimes, when older adults collapse due to a fainting spell, they may also sustain limb fractures. However, the actual cause of the fainting episode often remains unknown, and only the fracture is treated initially. Later on, it may become apparent that the fainting spells were caused by the undiagnosed Sick Sinus Syndrome or other rhythm disorders, which can also lead to fatal outcomes if left untreated.

When an older adult experiences fainting due to a low heart rate and sustains an injury, it is essential to consider the possibility of Sick Sinus Syndrome and conduct a thorough evaluation. The diagnostic tool for this condition is typically an ECG, but sometimes, obtaining an accurate ECG during the acute episode can be challenging as the patient may have already recovered by the time they reach the hospital. In such cases, further investigations like loop recorder or Holter monitoring are necessary to monitor the heart's rhythm continuously over the next 24 hours. Fluctuations or abnormalities in the rhythm, with very fast or very low heart rate episodes, may indicate a rhythm disorder. Correlating the timing of the low pulse rate with symptoms like dizziness can provide more clues for an accurate diagnosis. Thus, dizziness and fainting are often the first presentations of Bradyarrhythmia. If both slow and fast heart rates occur in Sinus node disease, it is termed the tachy-brady variant of Sick Sinus Syndrome, which is very symptomatic.

Moving on to the second type of Brady arrhythmias, AV nodal disease. The AV node, or Atrioventricular node, is the current transmitter for the heart's lower chambers. Sometimes, this node can become compromised for various reasons, such as congenital diseases, acquired diseases, or acute illnesses like myocardial infarction (heart attack), which may be transient or permanent. As a result, the heart rate can significantly slow down. For instance, the lower chambers may only beat twice when the SA node generates five beats. This imbalance can lead to symptoms like giddiness, syncope, and dizziness spells.

Unlike SA node dysfunction, where the AV node can adapt to the slower rhythm, in AV nodal disease, the rhythm between the chambers becomes highly unbalanced and unpredictable, even if the SA node is functioning normally. This condition is considered more critical and often requires aggressive treatment. If the symptoms of dizziness and fainting are present, the immediate placement of a pacemaker becomes necessary without delay.

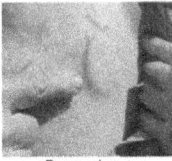

Pacemaker
Implanted inside
human body

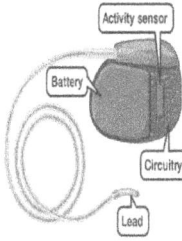

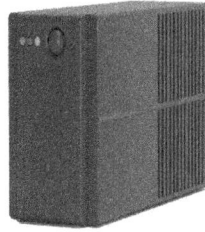

Best Inverter

Pacemaker- An Inverter of Heart

There is no medical treatment for AV nodal disease when the electrical conduction is compromised. The only effective treatment is the implantation of an artificial pacemaker. Initially, a temporary pacemaker is used, with wires inserted in the right lower chamber (right ventricle), and its wire is connected to an outside pulse generator(battery). Correcting an electrical emergency due to a low heart rate is temporary. The permanent pacemaker placement under local anesthesia follows it. The pacemaker provides the heart with the required electrical impulses, compensating for the compromised AV node. These pacemakers usually come with lithium batteries lasting up to 10 or 12 years.

The pacemaker is implanted with two wires connected to specific locations on the heart's right upper and right lower chambers. Depending on the diagnosis, only one wire may be connected to the correct upper or lower chamber. If a patient experiences giddiness, a temporary pacemaker is usually inserted first to provide immediate relief and allow observation before the permanent pacemaker placement. In certain reversible cases, such as increased potassium levels or an ischemia-like heart attack causing a reversible AV block, permanent pacemaker implantation can be avoided if the primary condition is treated effectively.

After the SA node and AV node, we have the left and right bundle branches. The slowing of electricity in these bundles supplying the left and right ventricle is called a left bundle branch block (LBBB) or a right bundle branch block (RBBB), respectively. When both the right and left bundles are affected, causing very slow conduction, it is termed bilateral bundle branch block or alternating bundle branch block. Once again, ECG is crucial for diagnosing electrical problems and providing valuable clues. Certain diseases can be ruled out if the ECG appears normal despite symptoms.

In heart diagnostics, ECG is the primary investigative tool for electrical diseases, like echocardiography for muscle and valve diseases and angiography for vascular diseases. Loop recorders are employed for cases where symptoms are intermittent or absent. These devices can record a patient's heart rhythm for five to seven days or even two weeks, allowing doctors to detect abnormalities during symptomatic periods. Modern implantable loop recorders (ILRs) are injectable devices that provide continuous ECG recordings for up to three years. They can be connected to mobile phones and the internet to remotely transmit vital information about the heart's electrical activity. These ILRs are invaluable tools for detecting SA node disease, AV node disease, or any compromise in the bundle branches.

Brady arrhythmias can have various causes and manifest at different stages of life. For instance, congenital heart block can develop in young children, usually around 5 to 10. This condition occurs when the electrical connection between the upper and lower chambers of the heart is disrupted from birth. Surprisingly, some children with congenital heart block may not display any noticeable symptoms, and their hearts can function relatively well despite the disconnection between chambers. Diagnosing and treating congenital heart block is not challenging but essential. A comprehensive evaluation, including valve and muscle involvement assessments, is necessary to determine whether pacemaker placement is warranted.

Some patients with congenital heart block may present during pregnancy. Interestingly, some pregnant women with this condition may not exhibit any symptoms because the slowing of heart rate is gradual, and their heart muscles are healthy and efficient enough to compensate for the electrical dysfunction. These women may remain asymptomatic even with a heart rate as low as 40- 45/min. This scenario also falls under the category of complete congenital heart block, and the decision to implant a pacemaker should be made after careful discussion with the patient and considering the timing of the disease.

Brady arrhythmias can also be acquired, and their causes can vary. For elderly patients, it is usually due to degenerative changes in the conduction system. The treatment approach is straightforward for patients with symptomatic brady arrhythmias, and pacemaker implantation is often the best course of action. However, for asymptomatic patients with AV nodal disease and a second or third-degree AV block, pacemaker placement may still be necessary to ensure a stable heart rhythm and prevent future complications. Pacemakers provide a lifelong electrical backup for the heart, maintaining a steady and regular heartbeat.

For instance, heart attacks can lead to a decrease in heart rate, resulting in brady arrhythmias. Infections like dengue fever and severe acute illness with electrolyte imbalances or acid-base disturbances can also lead to abnormal heart rhythms, including complete heart block or nodal dysfunction of the AV node or SA node. However, in cases where the underlying cause is treated effectively, such as reversing the heart attack or correcting the electrolyte imbalances, the patient's need for a pacemaker may be temporary, and the temporary pacemaker can be removed once the primary condition is resolved.

Bradyarrhythmia can be caused by various factors, including congenital, degenerative, and acquired conditions. Managing these arrhythmias requires a thorough evaluation to determine the best course of action, whether it involves pacemaker implantation or addressing and correcting the underlying cause. Pacemakers are crucial in providing electrical support for the heart, ensuring its proper function, and improving the patient's overall quality of life.

Tachyarrhythmia

Tachyarrhythmia, or tachycardia, is a rhythm disorder characterized by abnormally high heart rate. There are two main types of tachyarrhythmias: supraventricular and ventricular tachyarrhythmias. Supraventricular tachyarrhythmias originate from the upper chambers of the heart, the atria, or the AV node, which is also located in the upper part of the heart. On the other hand, ventricular tachyarrhythmias arise from the lower chambers, the ventricles. Within supraventricular arrhythmias, there are further subtypes based on their specific location of origin. Some originate from the atrial muscles, while others are activated through the AV node.

Paroxysmal Supraventricular Tachycardia (PSVT)

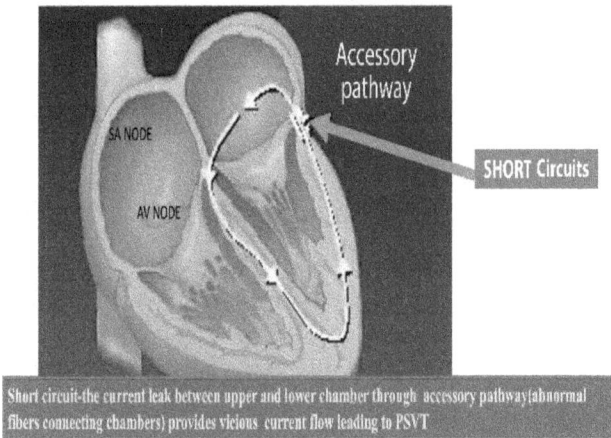

Short circuit-the current leak between upper and lower chamber through accessory pathway(abnormal fibers connecting chambers) provides vicious current flow leading to PSVT

> **PSVT (Paroxysmal Supraventricular Tachycardia) due to "Short Circuit" in heart**

A significant tachyarrhythmia among the Supraventricular Tachycardias is Paroxysmal Supraventricular Tachycardia (PSVT). It occurs suddenly when an abnormal pathway runs parallel to the natural AV node and bundle pathways, which allows current to leak from the upper to the lower chamber. This creates a vicious circle, where one pathway activates while the other recovers, resulting in an extremely fast heart rate. The heart may beat at 150 to nearly 250 beats per minute. PSVT episodes occur paroxysmal, meaning they happen suddenly and unpredictably. They can be unprovoked or occasionally triggered by substances like coffee, tea, or other factors.

To stop the weird heartbeat, we use a quick-acting medicine called adenosine. Adenosine works on a part of the heart called the AV node. It controls the abnormal heartbeat and breaks its cycle of it. Adenosine only works for a short time, about six seconds, but it's essential for treating the problem.

The weird heartbeat can happen in two places: the upper part of the heart (atrium) or the AV node. When it's in the atrium, it's called Atrial Tachycardia. This can happen if there's a scar or infection in the heart, making a part of it beat too fast, like the heart's natural pacemaker.

If the problem happens in the AV node, there are two types of fast heartbeats: AVRT and AVNRT. In AVNRT, the problem is inside the AV Node itself. In AVRT, an extra pathway outside the AV node makes the heart's electrical signals go the wrong way. In all these cases, there's an abnormal pathway in the heart that connects the top and bottom parts, sort of like a shortcut. This pathway might have been there since birth but only started causing trouble later. This messed-up pathway disrupts the heart's normal rhythm.

For Atrial Tachycardia, AVRT, and AVNRT, we commonly use the term PSVT (Paroxysmal Supraventricular Tachycardia). If the AV node is part of the tachycardia circuit, as in AVRT and AVNRT, we can administer adenosine, and it will promptly terminate the abnormal conduction. For all these PSVTs, an electrophysiology (EP) study and radiofrequency ablation (RFA) are effective treatments that can **cure** 95 to 99% of cases. The EP study helps pinpoint the specific circuit location in the cardiac chamber, and RFA deactivates them using controlled heat energy (RF burn), which is a painless procedure. This treatment can be life-changing for the patient, as it unhooks the patient from medication as well as from the doctor being a curative treatment for this arrhythmia.

However, medical management instead of EPS & RFA is preferred in young patients in their first decade. The procedure can be risky but still doable in selected cases when medically refractory. The manipulation of catheters in a very small heart can be challenging, and complications can have severe consequences on the heart's conduction system, leading to lifelong electrical problems. Because of these risks, EPS & RFA is typically reserved as a destination treatment initially managed on medication.

We prescribe medicines to reduce the frequency of PSVT episodes or stop them altogether. If compliant, patients may remain symptom-free for several years or even decades while on these daily medications. The decision to undergo RF ablation is usually made when the heart is fully developed, or at least when catheter manipulation becomes safer and more feasible, generally around 10 or 12 years old. By waiting until this age, we can minimize potential complications and ensure a safer procedure.

If a patient is not willing or not eligible for RF ablation, we commonly prescribe beta blockers like propranolol, metoprolol, carvedilol, or bisoprolol, as well as calcium channel blockers like diltiazem or verapamil. These medications help control the heart rate and prevent PSVT episodes. There are second levels of medication, like flecainide and propafenone, which are very effective if the medicine mentioned above fails but to be given under strict guidance.

EP study is an electrical study of the heart where we place wires, similar to catheters used in angiography, at different locations on the heart muscle to gather electrical data. It is usually done under local anesthesia or, if necessary, general anesthesia. After collecting the data and pinpointing abnormal locations, we can target and treat the specific abnormal points causing the tachycardia. This targeted therapy eliminates the problem within a small, specific heart area.

Atrial Fibrillation (AFib)

Besides PSVT, two other Supraventricular tachycardias occur in the heart's upper chambers: Atrial Fibrillation and Atrial Flutter. In atrial fibrillation, the heart's upper chambers contract irregularly and are out of synchrony with the lower chambers. On the other hand, in Atrial Flutter, a similar rhythm disorder occurs but with partial synchrony, resulting in regular and irregular beats that can cause symptoms like dizziness and palpitations.

Prolonged Atrial Fibrillation can lead to heart pumping issues, potentially causing a condition known as techy cardiomyopathy, where the heart becomes weak and may lead to heart failure. Additionally, Atrial Fibrillation can increase the risk of clot formation in the heart's upper chambers, specifically the left atrial appendage (LAA). These clots can be dislodged and travel through the circulation to various body parts, leading to conditions like stroke or other organ compromises, collectively referred to as thromboembolic phenomena.

Two main treatments address Atrial Fibrillation and its associated stroke risk. The first involves medical treatment aimed at preventing the occurrence of stroke. The CHADS (or CHA2DS2-VASc) scoring system is used to evaluate and stratify each patient's stroke risk. Based on the CHADS score, doctors can determine whether the patient qualifies for anticoagulant medications. These anticoagulants are oral medications and typically become lifelong treatments for patients with Atrial Fibrillation.

In the past, doctors often used medicines like Acitrom and Warfarin to thin the blood and prevent clots. But starting around 2009, there are new medicines called Novel Oral Anticoagulant Drugs, or NOACs. Some examples are Dabigatran, Rivaroxaban, and Apixaban. The great thing about these new medicines is that you only need to take them once or twice daily. And unlike the older medications, you don't need to keep getting blood tests (called PT/INR tests) all the time to check the dose. This makes things much simpler and more accessible for patients with Atrial

Fibrillation. Before, when people used older medicines like Warfarin and Acitrom, they had to be careful and get many tests to ensure their blood wasn't too thick or too thin. It was like a balancing act because too much medicine could make you bleed a lot, but too little could cause clots. The tests were essential to get the dose just right. But with these new NOAC medicines like Dabigatran, Rivaroxaban, and Apixaban, you don't need to worry about those tests. These medicines can keep your blood in the correct range, making things much more accessible for people taking them.

The newer NOACs have revolutionized anticoagulation therapy by eliminating the need for frequent PT/INR testing. Patients taking NOACs can avoid the inconvenience of regular testing and adjust their dosages independently, reducing the treatment burden. However, it's essential to note that NOACs are unsuitable for certain types of atrial fibrillations, and in such cases, older drugs like Warfarin and Acitrom may still be prescribed.

Lifelong anticoagulation treatment is typically prescribed for patients with a CHADS Score of two, three, or higher. Along with anticoagulation, patients also require rhythm treatment, which includes rate control and rhythm control therapies. Rate control therapy involves medications that control the heart rate and prevent paroxysms or intermittent rapid beating problems. On the other hand, rhythm control therapy is used when we plan to bring the patients into normal sinus rhythm. Antiarrhythmic drugs are prescribed in rhythm control therapy to prevent new episodes of atrial fibrillation and maintenance of sinus rhythm. DC cardioversion is often used to bring the patient into sinus rhythm. This cardioversion (shock therapy) can be done electively when the patient is stable.

In contrast, sometimes, when the patient is hemodynamically unstable or failed medical management, it is done on an emergency basis. On the other hand, the rate control strategy is enough when the patient is elderly and his hemodynamic, as well as echocardiographically good LV function but chamber size, is already increased, particularly of the left atrium or is associated with severe mitral valve disease, the possibility return to sinus rhythm as well as maintenance in sinus rhythm is minimal. Hence, a rate control strategy is best.

Treatment choice depends on the patient's medical profile, including factors like heart pumping function, coronary issues, and other comorbidities. Medications for rhythm control may be given for a specific period or, in some cases, prescribed lifelong to prevent further episodes of atrial fibrillation.

If the patient still experiences atrial fibrillation despite using these medications, the next tier of treatment is EP Study and RF ablation. During this procedure, specific burns target specific regions to reduce or eliminate atrial fibrillation episodes. This process is sometimes referred to as *pulmonary vein isolation (PVI)*, as the four pulmonary veins located just behind the left atrium are observed to be the source of extra beats that trigger atrial fibrillation. By ablating these areas, the abnormal rhythm disorder can be addressed effectively.

In the case of pulmonary vein isolation (PVI) for treating Atrial Fibrillation, the goal is to electrically disconnect the connection between the pulmonary vein and the left atrium. This can be achieved through two main techniques: radiofrequency (RF) ablation and cryotherapy.

RF Ablation: In this method, the regions around the pulmonary vein drainage area are encircled, and each area is treated with RF ablation to stop the flow of electrical currents in either direction(from the atrium to the pulmonary vein and vice versa). This process is called a bidirectional block, where it is demonstrated that there is no current flow between the Left upper chamber (left atrium) and the pulmonary vein that drains in the left atrium. After PVI, the chances of developing atrial fibrillation decrease significantly.

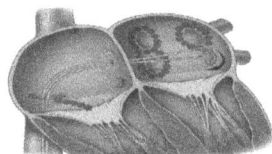

Radiofrequency ablation	Cryoablation
Better established	Simpler procedure
Less fluoroscopic guidance	More fluoroscopic guidance
More specialized training	Less specialized training

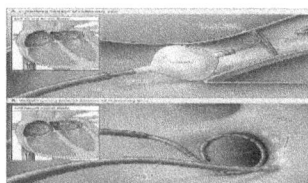

Atrial Fibrillation Ablation Method (Hot- RF Ablation, Cold- Cryo Ablation)

Cryotherapy: In this relatively newer technique, the regions of the pulmonary veins are frozen at extremely low temperatures (-40 ° to 60°C) for one to two minutes. This freezing process causes the tissues to necrose or die, interrupting the electrical conduction. Cryotherapy is an alternative to RF ablation, and both methods aim to achieve the same result.

Even with these treatments, some patients might still have times when their heart beats in a weird way called atrial fibrillation. If a treatment called PVI doesn't work, the next option is to do something more intense: they turn off a part of the heart called the AV node and put in a pacemaker. This is helpful for people who keep going to the hospital because their heart beats super fast (180 to 250 times a minute) during atrial fibrillation, and medicines and PVI don't work. This can make them feel bad and even lead to heart problems.

By turning off the AV node and letting the pacemaker control the heart's lower parts, the heart rate can go back to normal. This stops the times when the heart races during atrial fibrillation. This way might be better for the wallet in the long run because it can save money compared to doing PVI repeatedly. PVI may help a bit but not entirely fix the problem.

It's essential to know that all these treatments have risks. The PVI one can be tricky and take a long time, and it might not go well, especially if the doctor doing it isn't very experienced. There's also a tiny chance of getting a severe problem called esophageal atrial fistula. So, doctors usually only use PVI when they've tried everything else, and the person still has many issues because of atrial fibrillation. In summary, Supraventricular Tachycardias (SVTs) has three main variants: paroxysmal supraventricular tachycardia (PSVT), Atrial Fibrillation, and Atrial Flutter. PSVT is considered curable, with treatment options like EPS & RFA providing an effective cure. In contrast, atrial flutter and fibrillation are not completely curable, and treatment approaches aim to manage the condition, control heart rate, and prevent complications like thromboembolic phenomena.

Ventricular Tachyarrhythmias

There are two types of Tachycardias arising from the heart. One arises from the upper part of the heart, also known as Supraventricular Tachycardia. The other form of tachycardia occurs from the heart's lower half, specifically the two ventricles. This is known as Ventricular Tachycardia.

Generally, Supraventricular Tachycardias are milder and less life-threatening. While they can cause discomfort and symptoms such as palpitations and dizziness, they are *not usually fatal.* On the other hand, Ventricular Tachycardias are severe and potentially deadly. Ventricular tachycardia, ventricular fibrillation, or ventricular flutter can lead to life-threatening rhythms. Any tachyarrhythmia originating from the lower chamber can be dangerous because it immediately compromises the heart's pumping function as it originates from the conduction system below the safety valve of the conduction system and transmitter of the heart (AV Node). The heart may struggle to pump blood, causing a sudden drop in blood pressure, loss of consciousness, and, in some cases, death. Ventricular Tachycardia and Ventricular Fibrillation are among the most critical rhythm disorders and can be fatal within seconds to minutes. This sets them apart from other heart ailments, including heart attacks, which can also be life-threatening but often take longer to manifest.

The exact reasons why a patient develops Ventricular Tachyarrhythmias are not fully understood. However, abnormal genetic conditions can lead to the activation of abnormal electric channels that disrupt the normal flow of current in the heart. This channelopathy can involve various ions, such as sodium, potassium, and calcium, which play crucial roles in the conduction of electricity and the contraction and relaxation of the heart muscle. When these channels malfunction or become inherently abnormal, they can lead to channelopathies, which are conditions that often result in deadly Tachycardias or Tachyarrhythmias.

Long QT Syndrome is a common type of channelopathy that can lead to Ventricular Tachycardia. It is characterized by abnormalities in the QT segment of the ECG graph, known as repolarization abnormalities. These electrical abnormalities are often due to channelopathies that behave abnormally under specific circumstances. Long QT Syndrome has been extensively studied in the past few decades, especially in cases of sudden death in newborn babies during activities like playing or sleeping. The condition is genetic and can present in individuals usually under the age of 20.

Very recently, a 14-year-old girl visited us because she had quite a rollercoaster of experiences. She fainted three times. One of these fainting spells happened while she was getting her COVID-19 vaccine; the other was during a casual game at the playground. Adding to her list of challenges, she also had some trouble with her hearing. So, she came to us for answers. We ran some tests to figure out what happened. Her ECG and a gadget called a Holter helped us figure out what was happening. It turns out she had something called Long QT syndrome, a condition that can mess with the heart's electrical activity. We dug even deeper with a genetic study, revealing that she had a specific type, the Long QT 1 variant. Now that we've got a name for the game, we can work on keeping her heart and health in check. It's a journey, but she's not alone in this adventure!

If sudden cardiac arrest or death occurs in a family member, especially at a young age, there is a higher risk of other family members having Long QT Syndrome. This syndrome can manifest in both resting and exercise-induced states. ECG is the primary diagnostic tool for Long QT, as it can reveal clues of channelopathies that may not be visible in an Echocardiogram. Prolonged ECG monitoring with loop recorders can also provide valuable information, and in some cases, an Electrophysiology (EP) study may be necessary to identify any existing electrical issues. Provocative tests, where a drug is used as a stressor, can be conducted to assess abnormality.

Brugada Syndrome is another genetic disorder that affects the ventricle muscles and can lead to dangerous irregular heartbeats and Ventricular Tachycardia. This condition can be life-threatening, often resulting in syncope or sudden death, particularly during sleep or rest.

I once treated a 28-year-old, full of life and hope, who came to us with a mysterious problem. Three times in the past six months, he'd experienced fainting spells lasting 15-20 seconds. During these episodes, he'd stop breathing, go into convulsions, and then miraculously snap back to life. The weird part? He couldn't remember a thing about what happened. Worried sick, he'd already visited a neurologist who ran a battery of tests, including CT and MRI scans of his brain, an EEG (brainwave test), and even a nerve conduction study. To everyone's surprise, all these tests came back absolutely normal. It was like a puzzle with missing pieces. His journey led him to a general physician who directed him our way. It was time to dig deeper. We looked at his ECG and compared it to a previous one. That's when we spotted something that raised alarm bells – classical signs of Brugada syndrome. This syndrome messes with the electrical circuitry of the heart, and in this guy's case, it had led to three cardiac arrests, followed by some kind of miracle as he bounced back each time.

So, the next step was to implant an AICD (Automatic Implantable Cardioverter-Defibrillator) and give him some medication to keep that unruly heart rhythm in check. But the story doesn't end here. He had one more episode of chaos in his heart, a Ventricular Fibrillation, and this time, he felt a reeling sensation. But the AICD knew precisely what to do – it delivered a shock, and he stayed conscious.

This was the moment of truth. It sealed the diagnosis of this scary rhythm disorder (Brugada Syndrome) and highlighted the life-saving magic of the AICD. It's like having a guardian angel inside, ready to shock the heart back into rhythm when things go haywire. So, this is a reminder that sometimes our hearts can have a mind of their own, and having the right technology in place can make all the difference between life and something much darker.

In Ventricular Tachyarrhythmias with a structurally normal heart, diagnosis is typically made through ECG, with additional support from Echo and Cardiac MRI if needed. Treatment options include beta blockers and specific antiarrhythmic drugs to prevent future episodes and reduce the risk of Long QT variations. For the most effective and definitive treatment, AICD (Automatic Implantable Cardioverter Defibrillator) implantation is often recommended, even at a young age, to treat the life-threatening rhythm disorder.

Ventricular Tachyarrhythmia can arise from either channelopathies or abnormal circuits in the heart. Channelopathies involve structurally normal hearts, which may appear normal in an Echocardiogram, but VT occurs due to abnormal electric channels. The other type of VT happens in a patient with a structural heart where abnormal circuits are formed in response to injury (ischemic or inflammatory), providing nidus to reentry circuits (*short-circuit electrical pathways*). An EP study can help identify the source of the rhythm disorder; RF ablation can be used for treatment.

Specific types of VT are known as fascicleventricular tachycardia, RVOT (right ventricle outflow tract) VT, and LVOT (left ventricle outflow tract) VT. In these cases, certain muscle fibers in specific regions give extra beats, and EP study can pinpoint the region and facilitate RF ablation, potentially curing the disease.

However, VT can also occur in the presence of structural heart diseases, leading to a weakened heart pumping or enlargement of the heart chambers. In such cases, the treatment approach changes. Instead of RF ablation, device therapy is recommended, and ICDs (Implantable Cardioverter-Defibrillators) are used. ICDs can detect abnormal rhythms and restore normal rhythms by delivering ATP (Anti tachycardia Pacing) or providing shock therapy when it detect life-threatening rhythm, known as DF or Defibrillation.

Overall, Ventricular Tachyarrhythmias can be unpredictable and dangerous, and appropriate treatment options depend on the specific type of VT and the condition of the heart. In structurally normal hearts, EP study and RF ablation are viable treatments, while for structural heart diseases, device therapy with ICDs and antiarrhythmic is a more suitable approach to controlling and managing the rhythm disorder effectively.

When a patient experiences a sudden cardiac arrest and the heart appears structurally normal (regular Echo and coronary angiogram), implanting an AICD (Automatic Implantable Cardioverter Defibrillator) is the standard approach. The AICD helps to abort further cardiac arrests leading to sudden cardiac deaths by detecting life-threatening rhythms and giving the appropriate electrical therapy to bring the patient back to life. Sometimes, the patient continues to experience multiple shocks from the AICD due to active electrical problems. EP study must identify and modify any abnormal circuits causing the rhythm disorder. In addition to AICD therapy, medical management with antiarrhythmic medications may be escalated to better control the condition.

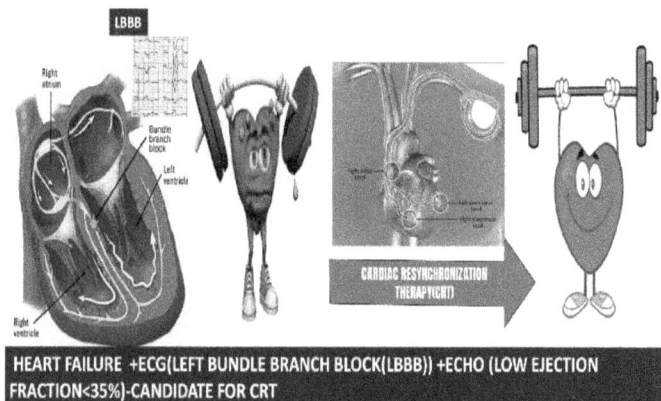

HEART FAILURE +ECG(LEFT BUNDLE BRANCH BLOCK(LBBB)) +ECHO (LOW EJECTION FRACTION<35%)-CANDIDATE FOR CRT

Cardiac Function Booster- CRT

AICDs generally serve as *"Z security to rhythm disorder"* in patients with or without structural abnormalities in the heart. However, suppose there is a specific abnormality like a left bundle branch block or a prolonged QRS duration on the ECG and associated weakening of the heart's pump function reflecting as reduced ejection fraction in the echocardiogram. In that case, an AICD may not be sufficient. Instead, a CRTD (Cardiac Resynchronization Therapy Defibrillator) is used. The CRTD is a more advanced device that improves pumping functionality and protects the heart from abnormal rhythms, similar to an AICD. Thus, CRTD works like *Z+ security* of the heart and is considered the final treatment option for heart patients with rhythm disorders caused by electrical issues along with heart pump failure.

When a patient experiences cardiac arrest with no structural abnormality in the heart, an AICD is often used for secondary prevention, which helps prevent future episodes of cardiac arrest. However, there are cases where doctors must decide between medical management and implanting an AICD. The old norm was that people with less than 35% EF (Ejection Fraction) should have an AICD since they might be more prone to rhythm disorders. But this is an oversimplification, and data are evolving that particular set of a patient who has either significant scar or ischemic cardiomyopathy patients have a beneficial effect, particularly if we are planning for primary prevention indication. That means if the patient has not suffered from sudden cardiac arrest or VT/ VF episodes, then carefully choose the patient. Cardiac MRI provides important information regarding the scar burden or structural abnormalities.

AICD placement as a primary prevention strategy (to prevent the first episode of cardiac arrest) should be carefully considered based on individual cases. Doctors and patients should consider factors like whether the heart condition is ischemic or non-ischemic, evidence of a scar in the heart muscle, and the patient's overall health. Placing an AICD for primary prevention without strong validation may not be the best option, as it can limit the patient's quality of life.

DR. ASHUTOSH KUMAR

11

HARMONY WITH DIAGNOSIS, DRUGS, AND DEVICES

"In the symphony of life, knowing when to heed the wisdom of experts and when to lend an ear to the collective voices of people is the art of harmony."

- Don Santo

Harmony in every space, whether a relationship or the workplace, is essential for healthy living. But it is also critical for disease diagnosis, and if it is incurable. Establishing a harmonious relationship is vital to prevent complications of the disease. For example, hypertension a disease of billion (1.3 billion people on the globe) has hypertension. Accepting the diagnosis and one or a few medications with regular measurements is enough to prevent heart attack, stroke, kidney failure, and many more complications. It is the denial of this disease, which is responsible for about 1/3 of deaths on the globe every year, directly or indirectly.

When you are diagnosed with heart disease, assimilating the facts about the disease and its lifelong company can be challenging, especially if you haven't experienced a critical episode or are feeling better after initial treatment. However, it's essential to heed your doctor's advice and diligently continue with medication, diet, and exercise to maintain your well-being. As mentioned earlier, physical, mental, and spiritual exercises are all vital during this phase to prevent or delay any future complications arising due to neglect on your part.

Paying attention to your heart and overall health and understanding why your body works the way it does can help motivate you to take better care of yourself. Our bodies are connected to nature and have evolved to work harmoniously with nature's patterns. That's why it's important to follow natural habits like eating at certain times, exercising regularly, and getting enough rest. Follow these natural habits for a long time to avoid developing health problems. While medicines can help with health issues, including heart problems, returning to healthy natural habits is essential for better long-term health and well-being.

Harmony with Cardiac Medicines

Patients are always concerned about the side effects. They often stop medications on-premises, and if they take these medicines, they will have side effects, particularly if they have to live long. Most of the time, their incurable disease mayn't be symptomatic, as in the case of hypertension, and the patient doesn't find a reason or consequence of the condition per se. Cardiac medicines undergo extensive clinical testing to ensure their safety and effectiveness. They are metabolized and excreted from the body, leaving no harmful accumulations. Modern heart medicines are targeted to specific metabolic pathways, addressing the deficiencies or imbalances in the body.

There are two types of drugs - short-term acting and long-term acting. Some drugs work on targeted organ receptors to replace deficient substances, like providing thyroid hormone when thyroid levels are low.

Time-tested medicines like Aspirin and digoxin have been in use for centuries. Before being approved for medical use, new medicines undergo rigorous testing, including animal studies and human trials. Since 2008, all diabetic medicine must prove their safety from a cardiac point of view through cardiovascular outcome (CVOT) trials before they can be prescribed for diabetes control. Hence, safety is a top priority, and any abnormality found during testing leads to the rejection of the drug.

Cardiac medicines are generally safe, and patients should not hesitate to take them, considering the importance of heart health. Since many heart diseases are not entirely curable, lifelong medication is often necessary to manage the condition. Regular consultation with a cardiologist is crucial to adjust the medicine and dosage according to the disease stage and the individual's response to treatment.

Treating heart diseases requires a holistic approach, considering the overall health and functioning of major organs in the body. Each patient's treatment plan may differ based on their unique condition and circumstances, and adjustments in medication and dosage may be necessary over time.

Harmony with diagnosis of disease

Once the doctors know about your problem, you must understand and accept that you have the disease. Ignoring it can be really risky and even deadly. The diagnosis means you're getting married to a disease. **And** if it is not curable and won't just go away on its own. It would help if you took action to make things better. Facing the reality of the situation and doing things to improve your health is essential. If you don't accept it, the problems could worsen and affect other parts of your body. So, it's best to understand the situation and start taking steps to get better as soon as possible. Any disease is a functional impairment of an organ system. It can be transient or permanent. For example, malaria or tuberculosis, which are infectious diseases, are transient, and here, a medicine course helps the body's immune system expedite the eradication of the bacteria from the body. However, the same applies to hypertension or chronic diseases of unknown causes. In hypertension, body blood pressure is reset to a higher level, which can tax the heart, kidney, and blood vessels (arteries) of most organs in the long run. Therefore, we must accept this and harmonize our relationship by taking medication, diet, and lifestyle modification. If we follow this relationship, most of the time, complications don't happen. When risk factors transform into diseases, they may initially manifest internally and later externally with certain symptoms. Unfortunately, these symptoms may be mild and easy to overlook or deny, especially in diseases like hypertension, diabetes, or coronary artery disease. Such denial or ignorance increases the health risks not only for the individual but also for their families and society at large. While overdiagnosis is a concern in the medical field, ignoring the disease poses an even more significant threat, particularly in India, where some individuals believe they cannot afford treatment. However, in many instances, it is this ignorance itself that they cannot afford, as the consequences may become severe later in life. Conditions like diabetes and hypertension can be effectively controlled if addressed early; otherwise, they may eventually lead to heart multisystem disease and its complications. Patients must accept the diagnosis and manage their health effectively through lifestyle modifications or appropriate medical interventions. Early awareness and intervention play a pivotal role in maintaining overall well-being and preventing the progression of diseases and risk factors.

Dyslipidemia

It is good that people know their cholesterol levels and want to control it with medication. Cholesterol is a waxy, whitish-yellow fat and a crucial building block in cell membranes. It is not as bad as it is exposed. The bad cholesterol (LDL) and its oxidized form are dangerous as they stick to the endothelium and macrophages' cell membrane and initiate plaque formation and its growth in atherosclerosis. Cholesterol also is needed to make vitamin D, hormones (including testosterone and estrogen), and fat-dissolving bile acids. Cholesterol production is so crucial that your liver and intestines make up about 80% of the cholesterol you need to stay healthy. Only about 20% comes from the foods you eat. There is a tight link between synthesis and absorption of cholesterol. The different fraction of serum lipid is reflected in the total lipid profile. These are important to understand. The higher the LDL, the higher the atherosclerosis and related diseases (CAD, PAD, CVD). Lowering the HDL again is also a risk factor for heart disease (CVD). We have a drug to reduce LDL but no drug to increase HDL. Exercise is meant to increase HDL. Estrogen before menopause is protective from CAD by keeping high HDL. All the medication that increases HDL has neither been effective in reducing morbidity/mortality of CVD nor are safe and, hence, discontinued in the past.

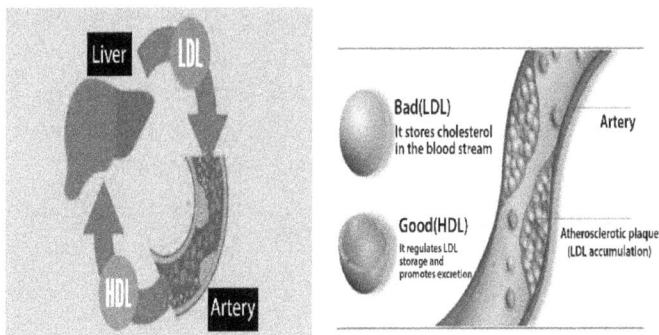

Cholesterol Journey from Bad to Good

1. Low-density lipoprotein (LDL) is the fraction of lipid particles rich in pure cholesterol as most triglycerides are removed in its formation. LDL is known as "bad" cholesterol because it delivers cholesterol to tissues and is strongly associated with the buildup of artery-clogging plaque. (Tissue cholesterol enricher).

2. High-density lipoprotein (HDL), the fraction of particles, is called "good" cholesterol because it removes cholesterol from circulation and artery walls and returns it to the liver for excretion. (Tissue cholesterol remover).

Understanding that cholesterol is more synthesized than absorbed from the intestine is essential. Hence, if you are having hypercholesteremia, it needs to be controlled, and you should know why it is a management target. There are two indications. Primary prevention is done when your cholesterol is high, and you have not had any heart attack. In these situations, we do risk scoring ASCVD as one of them. A score of more than 7.5% over ten years indicates lifelong cholesterol medication. The targeted therapy is fixed on the LDL level, but nowadays, the norm is the % reduction of LDL and achieving the LDL target level. A single value of LDL above 190mg% is marked as high cholesterol due to genetic reasons. Another family should be evaluated, and the index patient should be on lifelong cholesterol-reducing medication. This is all about the primary prevention indication of cholesterol medication.

When a patient has a heart attack, stroke (CVA), or any time revascularization (PTCA and stenting & CABG), any coronary block seen during angiography indicates lifelong cholesterol-reducing medication regardless of their cholesterol level. In this situation, we use cholesterol-reducing medication as a vascular anti-inflammatory medication rather than only cholesterol-reducing medication. Dietary modification helps reduce cholesterol, but remember that it is mainly manufactured and absorbed. Hence, it cannot be solely dependable to lower cholesterol by dietary restrictions.

Obesity

Rome was not built in a day, and so is obesity. It took a lot of effort to accumulate extra calories to be packed and saved in the storehouse of fat tissue without use. It is one of the most challenging morbidities to control than other. We should know what exactly obesity is. It is the enrichment of fat tissue with extra fat (fatty acid), a generalized body deposition. For every 1 kg of weight loss, 7700 calories consumption is needed, or 1000 calories is needed to be consumed for a loss of 0.13 kg. This mathematics is essential to remember. Do you know how many calories are consumed on the treadmill after walking/running for 30 minutes? In that case, you will be surprised how difficult it is to keep a negative balance to remove extra fat, which we have accumulated over the years. Your basal metabolic rate is essential, and lower BMR is responsible for high fat accumulation and obesity. This is one of the reasons why even non-foody become obese. Genetics is an important reason for obesity. The most essential ingredient in weight reduction is "persistence" and "willpower." Nobody has won over obesity without these two ingredients. So, it is essential if you want to reduce your willpower. Whether it is a keto diet or a workout in the Gym, they only give an initial boost in weight reduction, but long-term weight reduction needs a diet, exercise, and mindful eating habits. The hidden binge eating and habit of sweet (sweet cheat meals) are usually challenging to break and one of the reasons for the failure of weight reduction even after taking strict dietary restrictions and exercise schedules. We have no medication for weight reduction so far. All the earlier medication that has come into practice has been discontinued due to life-threatening side effects. Semagutide is one medication used for diabetic control and is showing promising results in weight reduction. It is used as an off-label indication for weight reduction. Bariatric surgery is the final resort for some patient who has failed by all means.

Hypertension (Disease of Billion's)

Hypertension, also known as high blood pressure, is a significant factor that can cause heart problems and even lead to a third of all deaths worldwide. Imagine driving a car and going up a hill, so you shift into a low gear. That's okay for a short time, but if you drive your vehicle in that low gear all the time, it's not suitable for the car. It will use more fuel, slow down, and wear out faster. The same thing happens in your body with hypertension. It's like your blood pressure gets stuck in that low gear, which means resetting it at a high level, which will tax your cardiovascular system adversely.

This puts a lot of stress on your heart and blood vessels. Over time, hypertension can cause various heart problems, depending on your genes and how you live. And it's not just the heart—it can also hurt your brain, kidneys, and blood vessels in your legs. All these problems are connected, and that's why controlling high blood pressure is so important.

Knowing about these risks and taking steps to control them can save many lives and make people healthier. It's like ensuring our "car" runs smoothly for a long time. Hypertension is the number one risk factor for death globally, affecting more than 1.3 billion people. It accounts for about half of all heart disease and stroke-related deaths worldwide. The global burden of disease (GBD) Study has estimated that hypertension led to 1.6 million deaths and 33.9 million disability-adjusted life years in 2015 and is India's most important cause of disease burden.

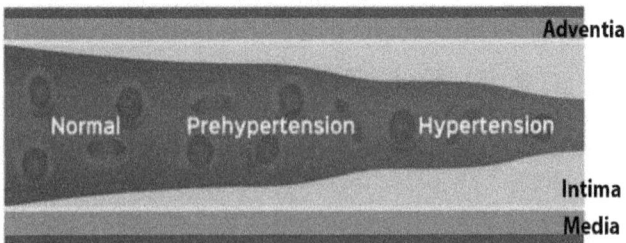

Changes in Artery during Hypertension

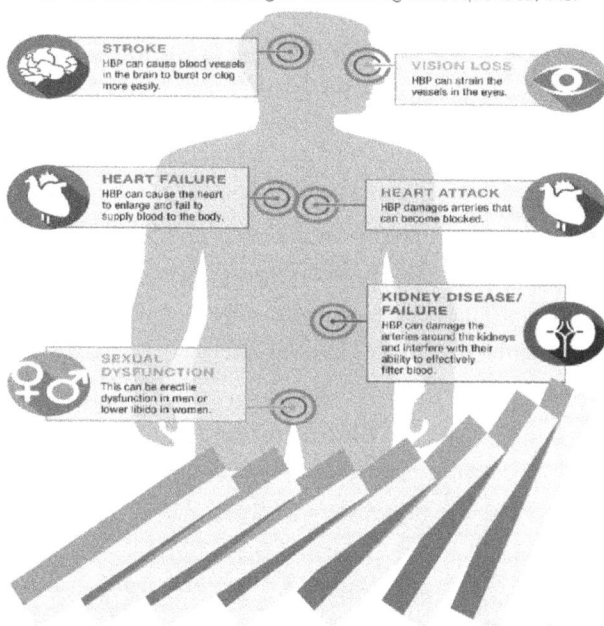

High blood pressure is often the first domino in a chain or "domino effect" leading to devastating consequences, like:

STROKE
HBP can cause blood vessels in the brain to burst or clog more easily.

VISION LOSS
HBP can strain the vessels in the eyes.

HEART FAILURE
HBP can cause the heart to enlarge and fail to supply blood to the body.

HEART ATTACK
HBP damages arteries that can become blocked.

KIDNEY DISEASE/ FAILURE
HBP can damage the arteries around the kidneys and interfere with their ability to effectively filter blood.

SEXUAL DYSFUNCTION
This can be erectile dysfunction in men or lower libido in women.

Consequences of Hypertension – Domino Effect

The permanently resetting blood pressure to a high level is mostly without cause (idiopathic) about 95% of the time. Addressing hypertension begins with non-pharmacological management, where patients must modify their diet and lifestyle. Restricting salt intake is crucial, aiming for not more than 5 grams (one teaspoon), which is equivalent to two grams of sodium. Foods preserved for extended periods are salt-rich, including traditional pickles, sweets, savories, ready-to-eat foods, papads, and fryums. Limiting such salt-rich products is essential. Additionally, physical exercise plays a significant role in managing blood pressure. Regular exercise improves vessel elasticity, reduces the load on the heart, enhances blood circulation, and acts as a stress buster.

Contrary to popular belief, medications are only the third aspect of hypertension care, particularly in critical diseases like cardiovascular diseases. While medication is essential to treatment, it works optimally with a healthy diet and regular exercise. These three pillars—diet, training, and medication—are crucial for managing hypertension effectively. Pharmacological drugs are well-established in treating the target illness, but their effectiveness is enhanced when accompanied by a healthy lifestyle.

Debates surrounding older versus newer medications and their side effects have often arisen. However, in the last two decades, advertising and marketing have influenced the discussion more than the fundamental differences in drug effects.

Blood Pressure Chart

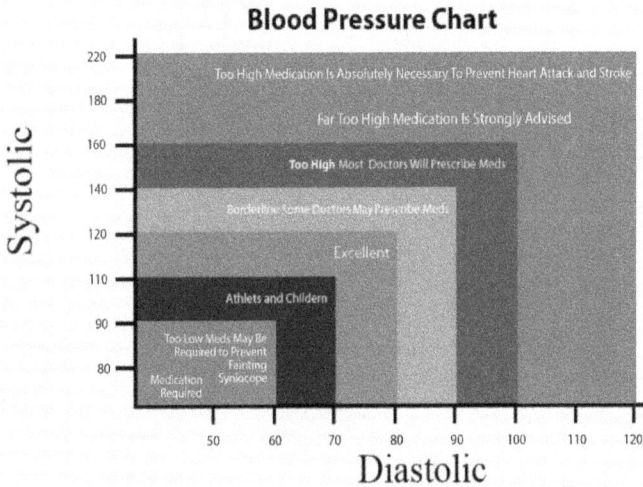

Too High Medication Is Absolutely Necessary To Prevent Heart Attack and Stroke

Far Too High Medication Is Strongly Advised

Too High Most Doctors Will Prescribe Meds

Borderline Some Doctors May Prescribe Meds

Excellent

Athlets and Childern

Too Low Meds May Be Required to Prevent Fainting
Medication Syncope Required

Systolic: 220, 180, 160, 140, 120, 110, 90, 80

Diastolic: 50, 60, 70, 80, 90, 100, 110, 120

Diastolic

Blood Pressure- Normal to Abnormal Range

Your clinical condition determines whether you have diabetes, hypertension, or other disease or risk factors, often in various combinations. Each individual's overall risk assessment guides the selection of a specific drug that may be more effective in their case and experienced doctors can make such decisions. The primary goal of medication is to reduce blood pressure, which takes precedence over competition between drugs and drug companies. While some differences may exist between medications, they are minor and insignificant. What truly matters is the cumulative effect of the three practices, diet, exercise, and medicine, in controlling blood pressure. The goal of managing high blood pressure isn't to reach one specific number because blood pressure changes throughout the day. Instead, we aim to keep it within a particular range most of the time. The idea is that the perfect blood pressure, like 120/80, doesn't stay the same. While you're sleeping, it could go down to something like 100/70 due to how our hormones work at different times. These changes are normal because of higher adrenaline levels when awake and lower when we're sleeping.

But in hypertension, there's a shift in these hormonal changes, even when we're asleep, causing higher blood pressure levels at night. Some people's blood pressure goes down at night but then goes up again during the day, and they're called "dippers." But if this nighttime dip doesn't happen anymore, they're called "non-dippers." If your blood pressure doesn't drop as it should at night, it could mean you're at risk for serious diseases, even organ problems. Unfortunately, these changes are often not caught in regular check-ups, making it hard to spot these problems early.

Kidney function may deteriorate in non-dippers, leading to nephropathy, which can be a starting point for more severe heart and renal diseases that are challenging to manage. If hypertension is not controlled through lifestyle changes and medication, it can start affecting coronary arteries, heart muscles, and rhythm, posing significant danger over time.

Regarding medications, the same drugs may only sometimes be effective for some individuals. Depending on the hypertension stage and your specific risk factors, you may need to switch medications occasionally. This is where your doctor's expertise becomes crucial. Your doctor can customize your medication regimen based on your blood pressure levels, risk factors, and any side effects you may experience.

If you encounter difficulties or side effects with a particular medication, your doctor will evaluate the situation and offer alternative options. Additionally, the dosing of medications may need to be adjusted over time. Sometimes, you may need to increase or decrease the dosage or temporarily stop medication during an acute illness.

Hypertension requires lifelong management, and it begins with adopting healthy lifestyle practices such as a balanced diet and regular physical exercise, complemented by appropriate medications.

Unfortunately, many people remain unaware of their hypertension and diabetes, which is picked up during the evaluation of other diseases or surgery. It is essential to note that hypertension, as well as diabetes, are relatively asymptomatic, and the notion that temperament fluctuates in hypertension is a myth than a fact.

Living with coronary artery disease (CAD)

The diagnosis and proper treatment of Coronary Artery Disease (CAD), where the coronary artery circulation is compromised due to atherosclerosis. There are a bunch of medications typically to be taken lifelong, including blood thinners, cholesterol-lowering drugs, and other supportive medications such as beta-blockers, ACE inhibitors, and ARBs (Angiotensin receptor blockers). They can markedly reduce the progression of coronary block, which is enough to live in harmony with this deadly disease, and if there is anything else, our body self-heals. Most of the time, by growing alternative circulation (collateral branches from the same blocked coronary artery or nearby branch, the body does its own" natural bypass," which depends on many factors, including diet, exercise, and genetics. The collateral circulation is decent enough to meet the requirement of heart muscle metabolism needed for pumping blood to the whole body.

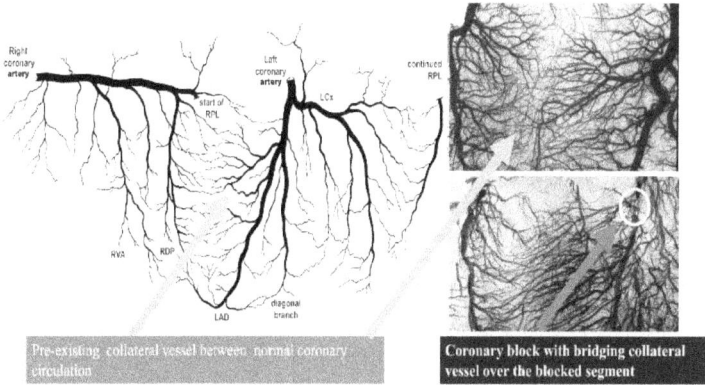

Pre-existing collateral vessel between normal coronary circulation

Coronary block with bridging collateral vessel over the blocked segment

Collateral Circulation- "Natural Bypass – nature to bypass block."

In cases where disease management becomes challenging and symptoms persist or recur, antianginal medications may also be prescribed. We now have many drugs, which include medications like Nicorandil, Ranolazine, Trimetazidine, and instant relieving medication like Nitrate(sorbitrate). Unlike the above medicines, these drugs help modify myocardial oxygen requirements to alleviate symptoms but not the progression of the disease. When we are exhausted with medical management, we can embark on interventional revascularization treatment procedures, including angioplasty and CABG, which provide a quick fix to the problem of the block. Patients feel better immediately after the intervention. A patient at high risk for intervention and still symptomatic on the above medication but not willing for intervention can take an opportunity of ECCP therapy, which also helps in selected cases.

As we have been discussing, coronary artery disease (CAD) is a manifestation of atherosclerosis, which is a lifelong disease. Once you have experienced a compromised heart circulation, such as in a heart attack episode, it becomes crucial to prevent future occurrences. Your next target or essential action is to focus on preventing another episode. This involves understanding that after experiencing a heart attack, you must take medications for the rest of your life, with only a few exceptions. The type or dosage of medicines may vary over time based on your condition, as assessed by your medical expert.

In the initial stages, if you have received a stent, there will likely be a higher dose of medicines to prevent the stent thrombosis in the initial vulnerable period and prevent the progression of any residual disease. While most of the healing occurs in the first four to six weeks, it usually takes three to 6 months for the vessel path and blood circulation to stabilize to normal levels. This timing is getting shorter with innovations in stent evolution and drug delivery.

After this healing period, to prevent the progression of atherosclerosis, we need to take measures to correct adverse remodeling, where the vessel tries to expand its outward layer, potentially leading to plaque rupture and clot formation. Medicines like blood thinners(antiplatelet) are crucial to the treatment and usually continue indefinitely.

By following your medical expert's advice, taking the prescribed medications, and making necessary lifestyle modifications, you can manage CAD and reduce the risk of future complications. Regular follow-ups with your healthcare provider will help monitor your condition and adjust the treatment plan as needed, ensuring you can lead a healthy and fulfilling life with CAD. Prevention and active management are vital to living well with this lifelong disease.

As I have emphasized, while medicines are crucial, exercise and diet form the foundation for managing coronary artery disease (CAD). "Exercise is a pill" and should not be missed. It should be initiated in the hospital, where the cardiac rehabilitation team will guide and advise you on the appropriate activities. Continuing these exercises after leaving the hospital is essential for maintaining heart health. The outlook may be more favorable if you reported to the hospital within four to six hours and received early stenting. However, if stenting occurred one day after the heart attack, some heart muscle compromise may have necessitated closer monitoring of symptoms and potential drug modifications. Awareness of these details is essential if you change doctors or need medical attention in the future, as it can help provide the best possible care.

There are limitations to angioplasty and stenting, mainly when dealing with minor vessels. If a particular blocked vessel is less than 2.5 millimeters in diameter, there may be better options than stenting. Attempting to place a stent in such a small artery could be complex and lead to further blockage. In such cases, medical management and lifestyle modifications, such as daily exercises and walking, can help the patient develop alternative collateral circulation, contributing to better blood flow in the heart.

A comprehensive approach to managing CAD involves a combination of appropriate medications, lifestyle modifications, regular exercise, and a heart-healthy diet. By actively participating in your care and adhering to medical advice, you can better manage CAD and improve your overall well-being.

Once again, the treatment approach remains the same as in hypertension, centered around the three pillars: diet, exercise, and medications, followed by intervention if conservative medical management fails.

Never forget that "Exercise is a pill," and its everyday dose may improve the effect of other pills or reduce pill burden and disease mortality.

Valvular heart disease and post Metallic Valve Replacement

A lifelong anticoagulant medication (warfarin/ acitrom) with target prothrombin time is measured as an international normalized ratio (INR). For most patients on metallic valves(St Jude, Chitra valve, Medtronic), the target INR is kept between 2.5-3.5 for the mitral valve, while for the aortic valve, 2-3. If the target INR is not in range, then a 10 -20% weekly increase is needed, and the weekly PT INR report is checked till we get the target range. If it goes above 4.5 and above with bleeding, dose modification is required in consultation with a doctor. A monthly PT INR of the patient is standard practice after valve replacement for a lifetime. Its importance cannot be ignored as it can lead to stroke or life-threatening bleeding emergencies.

For the bioprosthetic valve, we only prescribe antiplatelets after a short period of anticoagulant, except if the patient has other indications for anticoagulation, like atrial fibrillation with a high CHADVASC score.

Heart Failure as a Disease

Any heart disease can lead to different outcomes, including acute heart failure in heart attack and infection/inflammation(myocarditis). It may progress slowly, with gradual progressive heart disease presenting as chronic heart failure. A heart attack results in severely compromised blood circulation to the heart muscle, while heart failure is due to the progressive compromise of the cardiac pumping capacity of the blood, which can go downhill course before culminating in death if not treated well.

In heart failure, heart muscle pumping power is reduced, and it can be sudden deterioration during a heart attack and inflammation (acute myocarditis), or it may be gradually progressive over time (chronic myocarditis, valvular dysfunction). The heart muscles provide the pumping function of blood, and if part of the muscle is compromised or lost due to death or fibrosis, the remaining muscles must work harder to maintain circulation. However, they will not be able to contract as forcefully, leading to symptoms and potential complications. If left untreated, heart failure can eventually result in electrical compromise and cardiac arrest as a terminal event.

Heart failure is a lifelong condition, provided it is not due to reversible causes. The goal of treatment is to manage and preserve the remaining muscle mass. This is achieved through medical management, using medications that support the heart muscle and remodel it to reduce chamber size and improve pumping efficiency.

These medications and devices (CRT) placed inside the body under the skin work in tandem to maintain a healthy heart rhythm and pace. However, if medications and devices fail to meet the minimum requirements, a heart transplant becomes the last option for the patient.

Four main medicines are essential for managing heart failure: ACE inhibitors or ARNI, Beta-blockers, SGLT2 inhibitors, and MRAs. Doctors might give you a combination of these medicines based on how you're doing and other things that might affect your heart. As time passes, your doctor might change the plan if your condition changes. For people with heart failure and a reduced pumping ability, it's important to keep taking these four types of medicines to stay healthy.

Studies have used preserved stem cells regarding heart muscles and other organ tissues. Still, due to their complexity, they have yet to significantly succeed in regenerating the heart. Once the heart muscle is dead, it cannot be restored, and any damage is permanent. Patients must care for the remaining muscle for the rest of their lives.

Procedures like stenting or bypass surgery can help the heart improve with time, but the main problem that caused the heart issues, usually atherosclerosis, might still be there. That's why taking medicine for the rest of your life is important. The Four Pillars of staying healthy – eating right, staying active, taking medicine, and sometimes getting special treatments – will be important for your life. If you focus on the first three things, you might not need more special treatments, which is important for keeping your heart healthy.

Cardiac Arrhythmia

In cases of rhythm disorders or abnormal heartbeats (arrhythmia), there are two types. Some rhythm problems can be fixed entirely with special procedures and treatments like ablation studies with minimal risk of recurrence. The success rate of this procedure is as high as 95 to 99 in curing you if the diagnosis is paroxysmal supraventricular tachycardia (AVNRT, AVRT), which is excellent news for your health. When dealing with other rhythm disorders such as VT, VF, Atrial Fibrillation, or Structural Heart Disease, patients must live with the disease, and the role of medications and devices becomes crucial. Regular follow-up with an electrophysiologist is vital in managing the condition effectively. They can closely monitor symptoms, either orally or through device monitors, if the patient has an implanted device. Reading the cardiac electronic device (pacemaker, ICD, CRT) data requires specialized knowledge, making electrophysiologists the ideal professionals.

Harmony with Device Therapy

The heart is an incredible natural engine that's made to match exactly what our body needs. Its muscle mass, pumping capacity, and the pressure it creates all work together perfectly unless there's something wrong. Severe abnormalities can lead to acute syndromes and critical muscle damage, while milder ones can cause chronic and gradual muscle deterioration. In both cases, some heart muscle mass is damaged, leading to a condition known as Heart Failure with Reduced Ejection Fraction (HFrEF). This condition refers to a reduced ability of the left ventricle to pump blood into the Aorta, and the normal LVEF (Left Ventricular Ejection Fraction) range is between 55% and 70%.

When the ejection fraction drops to less than 40%, the first line of treatment involves medication using a combination of the four medicines previously discussed. If the patient's condition does not improve with medication, the second level of treatment is Device Therapy.

Device therapy entails implanting a device under the collar bone with wires inside the heart to regulate its rhythm and sometimes assist with pumping function as well. Patients can continue their daily activities with minor restrictions even after device implantation unless the disease requires specific limitations.

For people with irregular heartbeats like ARVD, Long QT

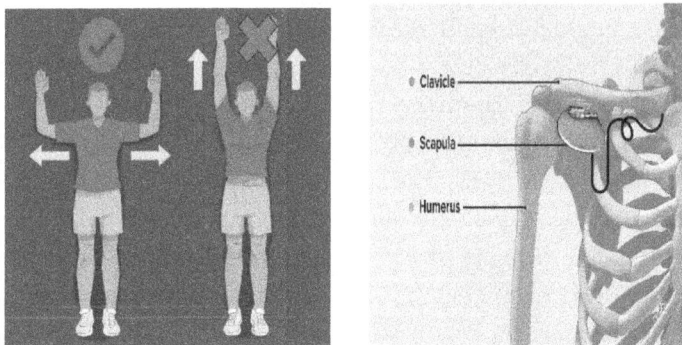

Subclavian Crush Syndrome

Syndrome, CPVT, or Hypertrophic Cardiomyopathy, it's best to avoid intense physical activities or competitive sports. These activities can trigger dangerous heart rhythms that may lead to a shock from the implanted device. So, it's important to be careful. Apart from very intense activities, they can live a mostly regular life. But we suggest they avoid lifting their arm above their shoulder on the side where the device is placed (usually the left side). Doing this too much could cause problems with the device wire, increasing the chance of complications. (subclavian crush syndrome).

The successful implantation of these devices relies on the expertise of the operating person and an understanding of the disease.

ICDs are usually implanted on the left side unless there are anatomical issues, as it requires less energy to convert life-threatening rhythm to sinus rhythm (normal rhythm). Additionally, most right-handed people can better tolerate the compromise in the above-shoulder movement of the left hand.

A distinction should be made between a defibrillator and a pacemaker. A defibrillator administers a high-energy electric shock to the heart during cardiac arrest. At the same time, a pacemaker provides the impulse to maintain a regular rhythm, for which it is programmed depending on the type of disease. The lifespan of an

ICD is typically around 5 to 10 years. In comparison, a pacemaker can last approximately 8 to 12 years, depending on its current consumption, which varies depending on the type of disease.

The procedure for implanting a pacemaker takes around one to two hours under local anesthesia, whereas an ICD procedure may take a bit longer due to its slightly larger size. These devices can be implanted in patients of varying ages, ranging from children of 5 years to individuals aged 95, whenever necessary. Age is not a barrier to device implantation; in some cases, even children may require these devices. The post-discharge patient goes home and can use most home appliances with few exceptions.

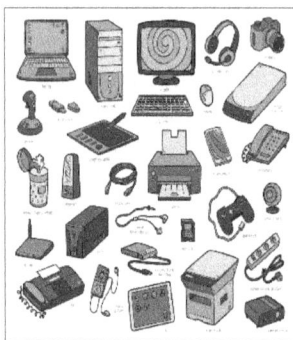

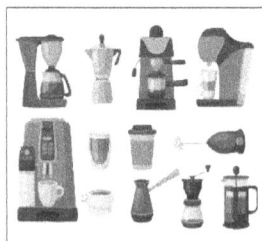

No Restriction for Home Appliances in Pacemaker and ICD patients

Typically, the implantation procedure is performed by experts or doctors specialized in electrophysiology, and these devices come with a limited global warranty of seven years. In India, four big global companies (Biotronik, Boston Scientific, Medtronic, and Abbott) make special devices for the heart, like pacemakers, ICDs, and CRTs. They are also known as CIED (Cardiac Implantable Electronic Devices). These devices help people with heart problems. Each company's devices work differently in terms of functionality. Let's talk about pacemakers and some important things to know about them.

First, there are two *types of pacemakers:* single-chamber and dual-chamber. The single-chamber pacemaker has one wire connected to either the upper or lower part of the heart, depending on the problem. The dual-chamber pacemaker has two wires, one for the upper part and one for the lower part of the heart.

Next, some newer pacemakers can even be used with *MRI* scans, a type of special test that shows pictures of the inside of the body. The older pacemakers couldn't be used with MRI because of some Ferromagnetic substances that could interfere with the device, but the new ones are made to work with it.

Another cool thing is that some pacemakers have *Bluetooth and home monitoring.* This means the devices can talk to a special system using your phone (if it has Bluetooth) or the internet. This way, doctors can check how your heart is doing from far away and advise if there's a problem. But remember, they can't control the device remotely; they can only see the information it sends.

You might need to pay extra money after sending a certain number of updates. This is good for people with regular symptoms so they don't always have to travel far to see the doctor.

Most pacemakers have 7 to 10 years of longevity, with global warranties typically covering up to 7 years. Higher-level or advanced devices may offer a lifetime warranty and require battery replacement every 7 to 10 years. However, it's essential to note that the warranty only applies to the device's Pulse Generator (PG) or battery and not to the wires or leads at any time by all companies. The patient must bear the replacement cost if any issues arise with the wire or lead.

Like Permanent Pacemakers (PPMs), Implantable Cardioverter Defibrillators (ICDs) also come in different variations, including single-wire, double-wire, MRI-compatible, non-MRI-compatible, and those with Bluetooth and home monitoring capabilities. ICDs are designed to address two main aspects: one for managing normal heart rates when the intrinsic heartbeat falls very low (bradyarrhythmia) by its pacemaker functions and another for treating abnormally high heart rates (tachyarrhythmias) that can be life-threatening by its defibrillation function. The ICD monitors every heartbeat and validates whether it is normal or abnormal. It takes action by giving therapy if it falls in the range of arrhythmia, which is programmed in the device. It is a miniature robot for rhythm management of the heart. It provides broad spectrum management of arrhythmia from bradyarrhythmia to tachyarrhythmia. In life-threatening ventricular tachycardia or Ventricular fibrillation, which can be fatal and lead to cardiac arrest, the ICD can deliver ATP (Anti-Tachycardia Pacing) therapy followed by DC cardioversion if ATP fails. This therapy involves sending an electric shock to terminate the abnormal rhythm and restore a normal heart rate. ATP is less battery-consuming and painless termination of arrhythmia, while DC shock consumes more battery and is painful; hence, it is the reserved therapy by ICD. Due to the higher energy consumption required for cardioversion or ATP therapy, ICDs are considered high-voltage devices, and their longevity is typically around five to 10 years. Companies may offer up to 10-year warranties or a combination of five plus three or five plus four years, providing discounts for later years. However, the specific warranty and replacement terms may vary between companies.

Cardiac Resynchronization Therapy (CRT) devices, which fall under the third level of devices, are available as CRT-P (Cardiac Resynchronization Therapy Pacemaker) and CRT-D (Cardiac Resynchronization Therapy Defibrillator). While CRT-P performs cardiac resynchronization with pacemaker functions, CRT-D incorporates both pacemakers with resynchronization of heart and defibrillation functionalities similar to an ICD. The main difference in CRT devices lies in using a third wire or lead for resynchronizing the heart during abnormal rhythms.

CRT devices are more complex than PPMs and ICDs as they require an additional lead to be placed delicately through the coronary sinus, which lies between the upper and lower left chambers on the left side of the heart, just above the left ventricle. This lead placement is crucial for CRT's proper functioning and requires high expertise. CRT devices aim to synchronize the upper and lower chambers of the heart and provide left-to-right chamber synchronization. The third lead is critical in correcting electrical rhythm, normalizing heart pumping, and addressing valve leaks or chamber dilatation.

CRT-P functions as a pacemaker with added resynchronization therapy, while CRT-D includes the same functions and the ability to terminate dangerously high rhythms through shocking. Like other CIED devices, CRTs can also have varying levels of MRI compatibility, Bluetooth, and Home Monitoring capabilities. Implanting CRT devices requires highly skilled experts due to the technical challenges involved; hence, it comes into the electrophysiology domain. Proper lead placement is crucial to ensure the effectiveness of CRT devices in synchronizing the heart's chambers and improving overall heart function. CRTs usually come with a guarantee of 5 to 7 years, depending on the manufacturer. Doctors typically suggest getting a CRT-D or a CRT-P device for people with a weak heart and reduced ejection fraction, depending on what's best for the person.

CIED-Device Upgradations & Replacements

After patients undergo implantation of CRTs, ICDs, or pacemakers, there will be a follow-up evaluation protocol for a specific period, usually three to six months. During these follow-up visits, doctors check the parameters of the leads, batteries, sensing, pacing, and other device functionalities. Any abnormal events recorded by the device are also reviewed, and modifications in the patient's medication can be made accordingly. This monitoring is crucial as these devices are typically used in patients with weakened hearts or ongoing rhythm disorders.

Several months or years after the initial implantation, the device may require either upgradation or replacement, which will be communicated to the patient. Upgradation is necessary when the patient's condition progresses from one stage to the next stage. For example, suppose a patient initially had a pacemaker that only treated low heart rates but later showed signs of a high heart rate situation that could be life-threatening. In that case, the device may need to be upgraded to an ICD or CRT. As for replacement, each device has a lifetime ranging from 7 to 10 years, depending on the energy levels it consumes. The device has a Beginning of Life (BOL), End of Life (EOL), and Elective Replacement Indicator (ERI). When the device battery reaches its EOL, it becomes a medical emergency to replace it immediately. The *ERI acts as a reserve mode* to avoid this emergency, similar to a vehicle. During the ERI period, usually around three months, the device company will notify the patient to replace or upgrade the device if necessary.

When replacing or upgrading the device, the procedure won't take as long as the initial implantation, as the existing leads and wires remain in place unless the parameters of the 'lead' are deranged when it may require replacement. The doctor will assess the device's parameters; if suitable, the old device or pulse generator (battery) will be disconnected and replaced with a new one. Patients can resume their everyday life seamlessly after the procedure.

Living With a Device

Living with a pacemaker, ICD, or CRT is not significantly different from normal living. However, there are a few restrictions to be aware of. Patients should avoid excessive left-hand movements above shoulder level and avoid magnetic fields, such as those found in MRI machines. Informing doctors and medical professionals about the device's presence is essential before undergoing any procedures involving magnetic fields or electrical therapy, including surgery where diathermy is used during operation. Devices like pacemakers and ICDs are made to handle magnetic interference, but when they're near strong magnets, problems can happen. The lead wires in these devices might get too hot and cause changes in how they work, which is not good. If a patient has wires that haven't been connected to the pacemaker (called "abandoned lead"), it's really important to avoid MRI scans because these wires could poke a hole in the heart and perforate it. If that's the case, doing other tests instead of MRI is better.

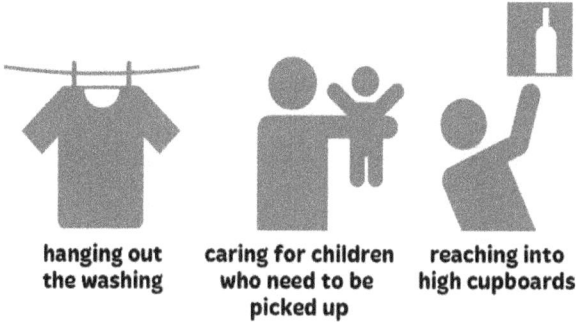

| hanging out the washing | caring for children who need to be picked up | reaching into high cupboards |

Home chores to be avoided in Pacemaker and CIED patients

Using things that need electricity at home is usually okay, but keeping things with magnets, like earphones, away from the implanted device is important. This will stop the device from going back to its basic settings. Also, avoid places with strong magnets, like security machines at malls and airports. If you let the people in charge know about the implanted device, it can help you avoid places that might not be safe. It's extremely important to remember the name of the company that made the device, especially in emergencies. Knowing the company's name is important if you need to get a new or upgraded device. Carrying this information all the time is really necessary. This way, doctors can quickly get the device's information and check how your heart is doing if something goes wrong.

- Magna-sleeps electric blankets
- Loudspeakers (must be 30cm away)
- Magnetic bracelets
- Electrolysis for hair removal
- Electric arc welders
- High power radar or electrical installations in close range
- TENS machines

> ## To be away from in CIED patients

Many patients forget this crucial information after a few years, which can delay necessary interventions during critical situations. Knowing the device company is as crucial as knowing your car's make, as it ensures timely and appropriate medical attention when needed. The PSA used for device interrogation will not interact with the implanted device if it doesn't belong to its manufacturer brand. These particular specifics make this point important to understand at this juncture. The hospital should have the contact information for the four companies providing these devices in India. Most hospitals do not have device clinics or in-house PSA (programmer) availability. Hence, they called the company to provide a device specialist to attend to it. However, it is not ideal to call all of them in a life-threatening emergency to enquire and match patient details to determine the correct device company. This issue often arises due to negligence during the implantation process, where patients or their families are not properly informed or provided with documentation and guidelines regarding the implanted device.

Hospitals and medical centers must take responsibility for informing patients and providing detailed information about the device and the company name. This avoids confusion and ensures that the patient and the doctor know whom to reach and procure the required device promptly during emergencies. Having the company name and other important device details, like carrying your

ID card, is particularly vital for patients with ICDs. In case of a medical emergency and unconsciousness, the data you have could be life-saving. Patients should also consider engraving this vital information onto a bracelet or another item that is easily carried and accessible in emergencies.

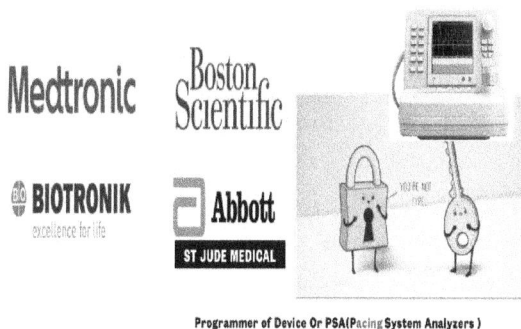

Programmer of Device Or PSA(Pacing System Analyzers)

> **Company Programmers can only detect your device**

Restrictions in patients with pacemaker and ICD/CRT

After having a heart procedure like putting in a pacemaker, doing a stent, or having bypass surgery, your body needs some time to heal, usually around four to six weeks. During this time, it's important to avoid doing anything too complicated or stressful, both physically and mentally. Once this healing period is over, you can gradually return to your regular activities. You can walk, jog, run, drive, and even play simple sports like catch. It's also okay to have sex with your partner, which is a healthy thing to do. Talk to your doctor if you take other medications that might affect your heart medicines. They can give you the right advice to stay safe and healthy. There are some specific restrictions for patients with device implants. Above shoulder movement of the left arm should be limited, especially in the first three months after a device is implanted. After this monitoring period, patients can resume most of their regular activities, but heavy physical exertion should still be avoided.

Professional drivers who have received an AICD (Automatic Implantable Cardiac Defibrillator are often barred from driving professionally due to the risk of ventricular tachycardia (VT), ventricular fibrillation (VF), or cardiac arrest, particularly in secondary prevention indication. These driving norms vary from country and guidelines. However, they may still drive their car for personal use. Patients with PPM (Permanent Pacemaker) and CRTs (Cardiac Resynchronization Therapy) usually have no driving restrictions, which may vary from country to country.

Doctors or expert teams generally monitor patients for three to six months after any implantation or acute cardiac episode recorded by the device before providing the green signal for a normal life with all regular activities. Patients are encouraged to clarify doubts with their doctor to ensure they can lead a healthy and confident life after cardiac interventions.

Heart failure patients, especially those using a device, may have marginal restrictions on their food intake due to their advanced stage of the disease. Limiting water and salt intake is crucial to managing the condition effectively. Generally, patients should consume less than 1.5 liters or one liter of water daily and keep their salt intake to a minimum (2gm to 3gm). Restricting fluid intake is necessary because excessive fluids can strain the weakened heart. The restriction depends on factors such as kidney function and the patient's environment and climate. Additionally, reducing salt intake helps control hypertension.

Regular physical exercise can also significantly support the heart, yet it is often overlooked. Exercise helps dilate the blood vessels, reducing the pressure on the heart during pumping. Therefore, exercise is a "beneficial medicine" for heart diseases, including heart failure, and a "health investment" for a normal heart. Patients can start with simple activities like walking and gradually increase the intensity over time. As emphasized earlier, a balanced diet and exercise are essential pillars in managing heart conditions, complementing the use of medications for optimal results.

Harmony with genetics (Parents' gift to the child)

We are gifted property and legacy from our parents, and so is the genetics. We are happy and feel proud after noting the movable and immovable property we have acquired from our parents and forefathers. Still, when accepting the gene-related disease, we start cursing our luck. Certain diseases, such as hypertension, diabetes, arrhythmias, and cardiomyopathy, often have elusive causes, with genetics and lifestyle being two recurring factors. While lifestyle choices can be modified to reduce risk, genetics plays a significant role in upbringing. In India, doctors only sometimes consider our genes when treating diseases, especially heart problems, where it's essential. We need more research because our family genes or new gene changes can cause heart and other health problems. Sadly, not knowing our family's health history can make people ignore these issues.

Knowing that your personality doesn't directly affect your blood pressure is essential. Checking your blood pressure regularly is important. If we don't control high blood pressure, it can lead to heart problems over time. Letting blood pressure stay high for a long time can harm our circulation. So, managing high blood pressure means changing our lifestyle, diet, exercise, and sometimes taking medicines. It's like a long journey that needs us to keep paying attention. If we get careless, our blood pressure can go up again.

When some women have high blood pressure (Gestational hypertension) or diabetes during pregnancy, it might go away after giving birth. However, the genetic risk factors don't go away and can return later in life. Women might be shielded from heart problems during pregnancy or between certain ages. Still, their genetic milieu can make them more likely to get heart issues during or just before menopause. Sometimes, genes can be behind health problems that don't have any other apparent cause.

Initiatives like UK and US Biobanks collect genetic data to study the genetic components that contribute to diseases like hypertension and diabetes, often leading to acquired heart diseases. While we can't change our genes, we can mitigate risks by taking better care of ourselves and modifying lifestyle factors. In health calculations, combining two risk factors can become a significant health problem, emphasizing the importance of managing lifestyle and genetic risks to maintain overall well-being.

Diagnosing a disease typically begins with discussing your symptoms and complaints with a doctor. A skilled doctor will conduct thorough symptom interrogations and further investigations to make accurate deductions. For instance, basic blood and urine tests can help confirm or rule out specific possibilities if you have any risk factors.

It's important to examine each person individually when determining health problems like high blood pressure. A skilled doctor will look at your medical history and the results of tests to understand what might happen. For instance, if someone has a family history of high blood pressure and strokes, the doctor won't just focus on treating it. They'll also consider how it could affect other important body parts, like the brain and kidneys.

Getting a clear understanding of what's happening is important. The doctor will advise on the best medicines and lifestyle changes to make. They'll explain how not following their recommendations could lead to more health problems. It's like getting a personalized plan to keep your body healthy.

Different family genes can manifest the same disease or risk factor differently. This highlights the significance of having a family doctor or physician who can develop a deep understanding of your family's genetic predispositions. Having a committed family doctor who can track your family's health across multiple generations allows for better and more accurate prognoses. This approach also fosters a strong doctor-patient relationship, reducing the commercialization of healthcare and ensuring more personalized and effective medical care.

12

RESETTING MIND WITH HEART DISEASE

"Your heart and mind work best when they are in harmony."

-Steven Aitchison

In the magnificent harmony of our human body, think of the heart as the nurturing mother, generously feeding and supporting every organ. At the same time, the brain takes on the role of the wise father, making crucial decisions for the entire system. These two, the Heart and the Brain, are like the dynamic duo of our existence, and their connection and teamwork are vital for our well-being, especially when dealing with illnesses.

Now, throughout history, poets and hopeless romantics have drawn these fascinating distinctions between the heart and the Mind. They've often assigned emotions and empathy to the heart, reserving thoughts and sensibility for the brain. But here's the twist: while all our ideas, even the mushy, emotional ones, originate in the brain, their impact on the heart and, consequently, our whole body is nothing short of profound. It's like a musical beat, you see. The heart's rhythm, the essence of our existence, can groove positively or get all out of whack, depending on our emotions and thoughts. Negative vibes, a grumpy mindset, and self-deprecating thoughts don't just mess with our hearts, but they also invite many other health issues to the party.

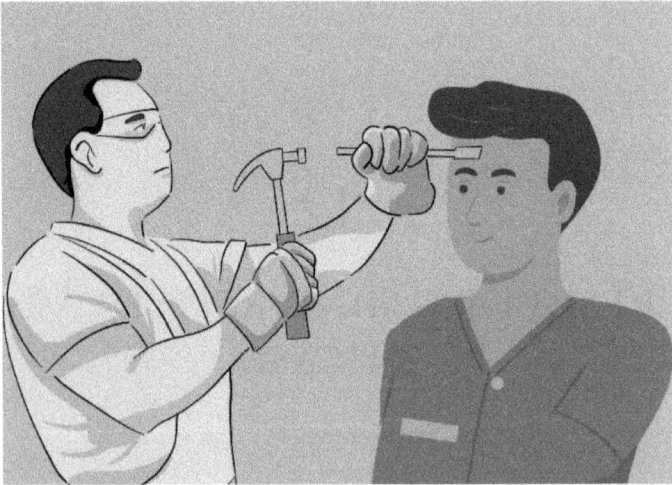

Suffering of Heart starts with the Mind

Suffering of Disease and Death

जातस्य हि ध्रुवो मृत्युर्ध्रुवं जन्म मृतस्य च |
तस्मादपरिहार्येऽर्थे न त्वं शोचितुमर्हसि || 27||

jātasya hi dhruvo mṛityur dhruvaṁ janma mṛitasya cha
tasmād aparihārye 'rthe na tvaṁ śhochitum arhasi

Bhagavad Gita 2/27-Death is certain for one who has been born, and rebirth is inevitable for one who has died. Therefore, you should not lament over the inevitable.

Let us be humble and accept the open secret that we are living in Mrityulok (means here who has taken birth has to die sometime, and the date, time, and place are already pre-decided). No one is blessed to be Bhisma (who has been blessed to die by his choice). Diseases are a Part of Life! Anybody who has taken birth has to die at some time; disease and accidents are modes other than Nirvana (for the yogic enlightened person who can leave their body by their choice). As we all know, the disease can happen to anybody, but sometimes it is caused by our habits and other times it can be a blessing from our parents through inherited genes. At the same time, we have a cure for a handful of diseases, mainly those from infectious backgrounds. Most diseases can be controlled by medication, particularly idiopathic and multifactorial risk disease, which has been pandemic nowadays, including hypertension and coronary artery diseases.

Resetting Mind- "Stop Shooting Second Arrow"

बन्धुरात्मात्मनस्तस्य येनात्मैवात्मना जितः |

अनात्मनस्तु शत्रुत्वे वर्ते तात्मैव शत्रुवत् || 6||

bandhur ātmātmanas tasya yenātmaivātmanā jitaḥ

anātmanas tu śhatrutve vartetātmaiva śhatru-vat

Bhagavad Gita 6/6 - For those who have conquered the mind, it is their friend. For those who have failed to do so, the mind works like an enemy.

Disease and injury are part and parcel of life. It is the first arrow that everybody has to face. How we face this arrow depends on our attitude toward life challenges. So if ever it comes in life, face it boldly! The pain of the first arrow, as described in Buddhism, is inevitable, comprising only 20 % of the suffering, but the remaining 80% is due to the second arrow. Think about it - no battle was ever won without a resilient mind and serious willpower. The same goes for dealing with diseases and setbacks. Life, my friend, comes bundled with the first arrow – pain and challenges. It's like the starter package. How you deal with this package depends entirely on your attitude towards these curveballs. The pain from the first arrow is just the tip of the iceberg, only 20% of the suffering. The real kicker is the second arrow we fire ourselves, mind you! It's our reaction, our storyline, and our worries that make things a hundred times worse. Sometimes, we're worrying about stuff that might not even happen – 85% of the time, to be precise!

Here's how you can look at it: The second arrow strikes the same spot as the first. Instead of doubling the pain, it multiplies it by tenfold. Unwanted things like heart attacks, accidents, or illnesses are like the first arrow. They hurt a bit. But the second arrow, fired by our thoughts, is where we make things messy. In this digital age, constant Google searches and WhatsApp messages add more arrows and blow things out of proportion. We often worsen the pain by letting our minds run wild with judgment, fear, and anger.

Resetting Thought - "Thoughts are Things"

मनः प्रसादः सौम्यत्वं मौनमात्मविनिग्रहः |
भावसंशुद्धिरित्येतत्तपो मानसमुच्यते || 16||

manaḥ-prasādaḥ saumyatvaṁ maunam ātma-vinigrahaḥ
bhāva-sanśhuddhir ity etat tapo mānasam uchyate

Bhagavad Gita 17.16 - Serenity of thought, gentleness, silence, self-control, and purity of purpose—all these are declared as austerity of the mind.

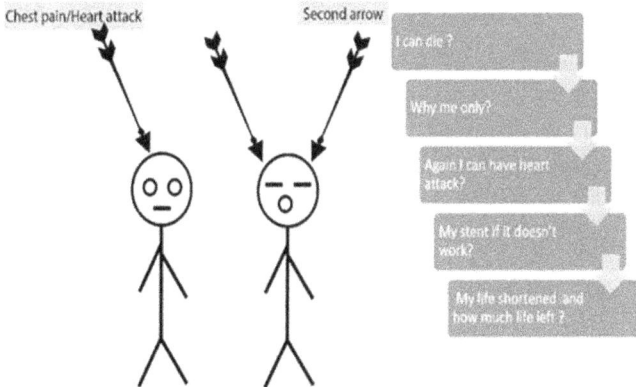

The Two Arrow effect and Heart Disease

The Mind is like an incredibly fertile soil. It will abundantly return whatever you plant into it. Our thoughts are like crops in the garden of our minds. Positive ones are like fertile soil for our well-being; negative, toxic ones are like weeds that sabotage our health. If we let thoughts of resentment, hate, blame, criticism, and condemnation grow wild, they can seriously mess with our health. So, keep an eye on your thoughts – mental hygiene is as crucial as physical hygiene!

And remember, water is a big deal in our bodies. Up to 60% of us are made up of this precious liquid. Now, our thoughts can affect this water content. It's been studied under a microscope, and it's a real thing. So, let's be mindful of the thoughts we're watering our inner garden with! Positive ones can help us thrive, just as negative ones can dehydrate us.

In his experiment, a Japanese scientist, Masaru Emoto (writer of the famous book-"The Hidden Messages in Water"), showed the influence of our thoughts, words, and feelings on water molecules. In his studies, Emoto found that water exposed to positive words and intentions formed beautiful, symmetrical crystalline structures when frozen. In contrast, water exposed to negative words and intentions began disorganized, asymmetrical structures. We talk higher with ourselves than anybody else. Hence, our thoughts and self-talk significantly impact our health and recovery during disease. What we are brooding in our brain as self-talk can significantly impact our health and disease. Hence, the mindfulness of our thoughts is essential in recovery from illness.

Resetting Emotion

We all know that the immune system responds to the antigen. But don't be surprised that "emotion" can also turn the immune system and lead to chronic inflammation. Our immune system is connected to emotion, thought, and belief and can be modified positively and negatively. A scientific basis is described in psychoneuroimmunity (PNI) modulation. Bidirectional communication occurs between the nervous, immune, and endocrine (hormone) systems.

The field of Psychoneuroimmunology has already provided information on how deeply our thoughts and our physiology are connected. No doubt, they will not take the headlines as the promotion of any investment in drugs or technology does not back them. It has been learned from many research that creating healing imagery with our thoughts can improve factors like blood pressure, inflammation, and immune markers, which have a role in healing. But as science advances our understanding of the mind-body connection, we find that the mind can influence our physiology and be a powerful healing tool. There is a scientific basis for it. Psychological stress has long been thought of as an essential human malady. Stress prompts activation of the sympathetic nervous system and the hypothalamic–pituitary–adrenal axis, leading to increased circulating catecholamines, glucocorticoids, and (eventually) inflammatory cytokines.

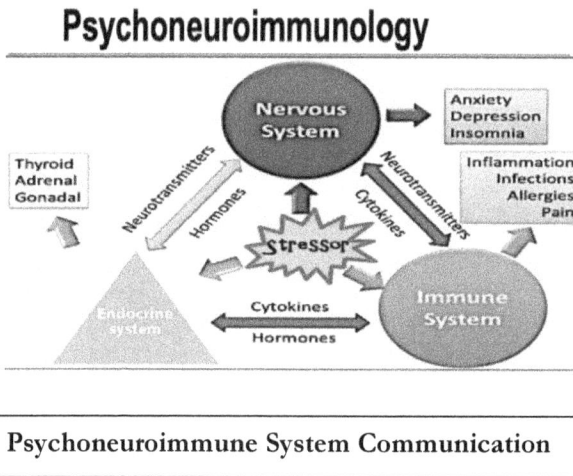

Psychoneuroimmune System Communication

Additionally, stress can increase heart rate and blood pressure via the autonomic nervous system, all of which can contribute to endothelial dysfunction (the first step in the story of atherosclerosis). A paper published in the Lancet by Tawakol Ahmed in 2017 showed how stress affects the amygdala through functional MRI and the progression of vascular inflammation (atherosclerosis) and cardiovascular events. Constant negative emotions and anxiety have a significant impact on our cardiovascular system. Resetting our emotional environment is as important as taking medicine and other lifestyle modifications. Positive thoughts and emotions help reduce the progression of atherosclerosis by inhibiting the amygdala and activating the immune system.

A study of a 12-week stress-reduction course experienced an approximately 50% reduction in cardiovascular disease events over a median follow-up period of 3.2 years compared with individuals who underwent cardiac rehabilitation but not stress management training.

Hence, with the discussed case of heart failure, you can understand how emotional baggage can affect normal recovery even with the proper medication.

Resetting Eye and Ear - Gateway to Amygdala

सर्वकर्माणि मनसा संन्यस्यास्ते सुखं वशी |

नवद्वारे पुरे देही नैव कुर्वन्न कारयन् || 13||

sarva-karmāṇi manasā sannyasyāste sukhaṁ vaśhī

nava-dvāre pure dehī naiva kurvan na kārayan

Bhagavad Gita 5.13 - The embodied beings who are self-controlled and detached reside happily in the city of nine gates free from thoughts that they are the doers or the cause of anything.

Our body is considered a temple with nine gates and seven on the face (2 eyes, two ears, two nostrils, one mouth), with God (Self) staying in the temple. We are very cautious nowadays while drinking water and maintaining food hygiene. We want it to be clean and healthy in all aspects. How many times are we cautious while ingesting the audible and visual content? Currently, "your attention" is currency, and the tech world (Facebook, WhatsApp, Instagram, Reel, Shorts, etc.) want to encash it by every means- your eyes and ear are now a source to get this currency.

The fear of death has been propagated in society with many methods, starting with mass media news feeds through this tech world. The truth of life needs to be looked at from a new angle; though I am not meant to discuss it, it is still essential to delve into death. We all know that "death" and "change" are universal truths. But fear has been created to hook us for some purpose. Let us understand why negative news and fear of death have been propagated so rampantly, particularly cardiac death. Bad is more potent than good to hook. We all have a negative bias, the tendency to get hooked more easily than positive information. As the writer said, the author has given a sound basis for thinking fast and slow.

We all are more worried about preventing a loss than about gaining. Our negative base has been ingrained for survival as a reptilian brain response. The Target Rating Points (TRPs) of a news channel go up by the channel's viewership. This hooking is easier with negative news than positive news. And when it comes to health-related domains, it catches fire. It takes the most attention, has a higher viewership, and is forwarded by WhatsApp and other means. The reason is simple. Health-related matters, such as sudden or cardiac death in young people, will always give a lot of discussion and viewership. The healthcare industry never leaves the opportunity to propose its package and cutting-edge technology to encash the situation. Everybody has read the news of sudden death and interpretation as coronary block driving heart attack due to exercise. Here, exercise is the culprit, and the unevaluated coronary block is the reason for sudden death in these young patients. The fact is otherwise, most of the time. A postmortem is needed to conclude the cause. If a person dies, there are three angles- chance, trigger, and cause of death. When we are living, we don't know what the life force is and from where it comes. We characterize it and accept it as life when it is in our body. But what is present as "life" and what is left from the body to define as death is not explained anywhere in science and never will be explained by science. But we have answers about when, why, and how it has left the body with exact timing. It comes under the domain of forensic medicine. When a celebrity dies or any unnatural death happens, conducting a postmortem to determine the cause is essential. Even as doctors, we often get surprises, what we have thought, and what has emerged after forensic evaluation. The recent sensationalization of the death of a celebrity either in the Gym or exercising provides a TRP to the channel. It produces a ripple of uncertainty in society, which should be avoided for the sake of public health. And the worst part of making a causal link (cause of death) of exercise to the death. Every death should be looked at from three angles: chance, trigger, or cause of the event. A well-conducted postmortem is the answer to diffuse the fear factor created by the sudden death and uncertainty in society. The sensational and causal association of exercise and Gym death has driven more business to hospitals and diagnostic Centers and improved the TRP of the channel. Still, it is a dishonest service to the viewer and society.

Let's accept that sudden cardiac death (SCD) incidence and prevalence have not reduced in the past few decades. Even though we have cutting-edge technology and the most advanced treatments, we have not been able to reduce the incidence or Prevalence of SCD even by a dot percentage. The risk factors of sudden cardiac death/cardiac arrest and heart attacks are similar. Still, the window of opportunity to act and revive the person is very short. It is in "minutes". A diagnosis to treatment in a public place is remote when it happens. That's why making a causal link between sudden death and exercise is fallacious. Why the person who exercised every day for years died only that particular day during exercise is unknown. This is also challenging to answer. It does not come in the realm of science to provide all explanations. Science has its limitations, and we must accept it at some level. The sudden death of a person needs postmortem and reporting to help society and not give information, which provides uncertainty, drives fear in the community, and builds business for the health industry. Hence, it is essential to keep hygiene not only of food and water taken by mouth but also of the content served to the ear and eye. Do not lose the currency of attention through eye and ear by digital burglars. The unhygienic content feeding through our eyes and ears to the brain, particularly the amygdala, will affect our health adversely. So, be mindful of the content presented to your eyes and ears. It is the most significant nuisance and can be considered junk eating by ear and eyes.

Resetting Purpose - "Journey from Head to the Heart"

When we are diagnosed with heart disease or chronic disorder, we are immediately surrounded with a lot of negativity and information about the complications of the disease as well as the side effects of the medication. We start living in a world of fear and uncertainty of our life. We were in the pandemic, and we are still in the coronavirus era, never forget the blessing, healing power of the body, and most importantly, your attitude towards life in difficult situations and challenges. Diseases are destined to come into our lives. It can compromise our physical function temporarily or sometimes permanently. But never underestimate how your willpower and attitude can make a difference. A positive attitude and resolve to come back reduces the suffering of disease and helps heal the injury caused by disease. I will strongly recommend reading the book Men in Search of Meaning. This book was written when we did not have good healthcare technology. A doctor has studied the person who survived the Nazi concentration camp and the Holocaust of the second world war. The physical, mental, and psychological challenge which you and I cannot imagine had been imposed on these prisoners. Their attitude and Purpose defined the survival of the prisoners. Those who have lost their family member and have no purpose died, while those who have a goal to live or meet their son, daughter, spouses, and parents, including the writer himself, can bear the challenges and survive. Hence, keeping your positive spirit and higher Purpose will no doubt help you tide over the acute health crisis but "work like medicine" when you have to live with diseases that are sometimes incurable and lifelong.

"Everything can be taken from a man but one thing: the last of the human freedoms—to choose one's attitude in any given set of circumstances, to choose one's own way."

— Viktor E. Frankl, Man's Search for Meaning

Any disease that comes during life causes suffering for a while, but it allows traveling the longest journey from the Mind to the heart. We often live within our thoughts, judging and perceiving life through this lens. While this feels safe, it limits us from fully experiencing life. To re-engage with life:

1. Shift from the head to the heart.

2. Recognize the stories and meanings you attach to experiences without judgment.
3. Embrace affectionate awareness, replacing negative thoughts with positive, inspiring ones. Life becomes easy, even difficult, as we align with our heart space.

When you get married to any incurable disease, knowing what you want from life is essential, not what others want from you. Following your passion and the work you love will give you freedom and an offload from the stress of what you are carrying out that you don't like. It is the time to reset relationships, workplace, and family life in a new way. Balance it well and excel in the field. Diagnosing the disease is the turning point to understanding the imbalance in life and correcting it or harmonizing it.

Resetting by Nature

Nature is like the ultimate healer, which has always got our back, quietly patching up the little bumps and bruises we accumulate daily without even sending us a memo. But you know what? It's not just about nature doing its magic in the background; it's about our relationship with it. Living close to nature is like a secret recipe for good health, a little thing they call "Ikigai." So, what's "Ikigai," you ask? It's like your reason for getting out of bed in the morning, your passion, your Purpose. Now, Ikigai is more than just a word; it's the heart of this fantastic book. This book is like a vault to the secrets of living up to a hundred and beyond! The authors took a deep dive into the lives of folks who've reached the impressive milestone of being a century old or older. They wanted to figure out what makes these superhumans tick. What they found was incredible. These centenarians, supercentenarians, and real-life legends all had a few things in common. It wasn't just a stroke of luck; it was their way of living. They engaged in physical and mental exercise, like brushing their teeth, as part of their daily routine. But that's not all; they were like friendship champions, always nurturing those connections, and they had this special bond with nature like they were best buddies. And here's the common thread – they were all following their "ikigai." These centenarians knew what made them tick and what got their hearts racing, and they chased that dream like a pot of gold at the end of the rainbow. So, what is the recipe for a long and healthy life? Daily exercise, good friends, a dash of nature, and a heaping helping of Ikigai – that's the ultimate secret! So far, all the resetting needed our intervention, but this resetting happened independently. We should avoid disturbing it by acting on the abovementioned factors. Many of us are fans of the superhero Wolverine from the hit action movie franchise of the same name. Wolverine has an extraordinary power. He can recover from any injury within seconds. We don't have powers like the Wolverine, but our body has a natural healing mechanism. So, in reality, we all can recover, not in seconds, but in days or months if the injury is severe. Every creature on this earth has an inbuilt repair mechanism. Our whole intestine's internal lining, called mucosa, is replaced every 5 days. Different tissues and organs have different timing. The human body has its own healing process whenever there is a subtle injury, whether internal or external. Unless the injury ultimately damages an organ or tissue, most of the time, a compensatory mechanism, which may be adaptive or maladaptive, takes over work while the repairing process is ongoing. For example, suppose a person develops hypertension, which we call *hypertension de novo*. In that case, the vessel muscle layer called media starts thickening to withstand the raised pressure, and its stiffness increases. At the same time, the heart also has to work harder to push the blood into these arteries, making it thicker, which we call cardiac hypertrophy in medical terminology. These are adaptive changes but, in the long term, lead to functional impairment of the organ. That is why we say hypertension is a lifelong disease and let us modify the illness with drugs, exercise, and diet to prevent maladaptation, which sets in when the patient develops hypertension. There are two common ways in which the healing process in the human body works. Suppose one has CVA (stroke) and is disabled briefly. You may see the same person start walking after some time, except in some exceptional situations. This is all due to neuron plasticity. The other side of the brain takes over the function and provides a compensatory mechanism. It is like one partner helping out the other partner in times of need, just like it happens in a family. Similarly, when a patient with risk factors like diabetes, hypertension, lipid problems, or genetics experiences the progression of coronary artery stenosis (block) due to smoldering vascular inflammation known as atherosclerosis, the heart responds by generating new vessels called collateral circulation. These vessels act as a natural bypass, assuming the patient maintains a high level of physical activity. These compensatory mechanisms again help the patient to survive even amid coronary block. Most organs in our body either get repaired or compensated through an alternative mechanism. Even in our body, there is a mechanism to eliminate abnormal cells. Wherever there is a damaged or abnormal cell, our body is brilliant in identifying it. It creates an inflammation around it and starts the repair procedure. Whether it's an external wound on the skin or a cancerous cell inside the body. Ideally, the immune system will detect and eliminate those abnormal cells. It becomes easy for the body to perform this task when people are fasting. It doesn't have to do a lot of tasks that it does otherwise, so it initiates a self-cleaning process to eliminate abnormal cells.

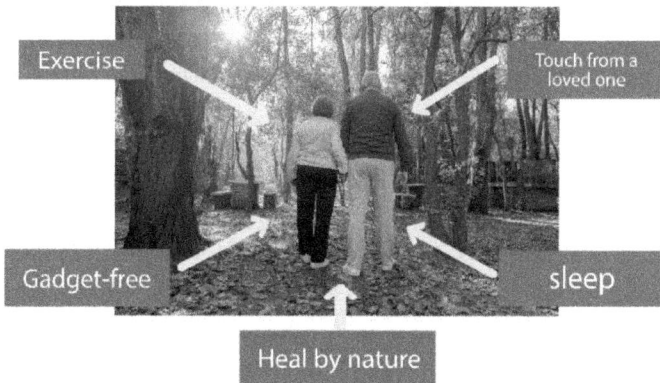

Non-medical Anti-inflammatory method to heal disease

Our body's cleanup crew is a fantastic body mechanism called *"Autophagy"*. When you've got some damaged or old cells hanging around, ones that might be thinking about turning into troublemakers (we're looking at you, cancer cells), autophagy steps in.

Here's how it works: Autophagy is like hitting the Reset button for your body. It's a natural process where your body clears out those worn-out cells to make room for fresh, shiny, healthy ones. It's like a mini-spring cleaning inside your cells. Now, here's where things get interesting. During this cleanup, your body isn't just tossing out the trash; it's also recycling. It takes the parts from the old, junky cells and uses them in the new ones. It's like the ultimate in sustainable living but on a cellular level! So, what's the deal with fasting and autophagy? Fasting, especially for around 14 to 18 hours, is like giving your body a gentle nudge, saying, "Hey, it's time for some cleaning!" Fasting is like the stressor that kicks autophagy into high gear.

The cool part is that autophagy has some serious anti-aging superpowers. It breaks down the old and busted cellular material and recycles it for all the essential processes in your body. In simpler terms, it's like your body's way of hitting the refresh button. This is why fasting is often linked to healthy cellular renewal.

So, if you're into feeling and looking your best for the long haul, consider giving autophagy a helping hand with innovative fasting. It's like your body's secret weapon for staying youthful and thriving.

To summarise this: It's not just those sneaky viruses and bacteria or those mysterious "risk factors" that can mess with our health. Nope, it's also the baggage we carry in our minds, the negativity that likes to set up camp. See, illness isn't just about germs and genes; it's also about what's cooking in our thoughts. When we hang on to those negative vibes, it's like we're inviting trouble right in through the front door of our well-being. So, remember that our mental state plays a significant role in the whole health equation!

As humans, our developed brains have blessed us with the most advanced creatures on earth. We share common behaviors, such as most animals eating, sleeping, procreation, and even fear. There is one difference- the ability to control all of these by its "intellect" gifted to human by God that pull human above all creatures on earth. The human brain's cerebral cortex, which is responsible for the higher cognitive capacity, is disproportionately large, accounting for more than 80% of total brain mass. In contrast, the cerebral cortex of the animal brain is not significantly larger.

The amygdala, or as some folks call it, the "smoke detector" of the brain, is a little powerhouse in charge of sniffing out fear and getting us ready for action when things get dicey. Let's say you're walking in the woods and spot something that looks like a bear. Your amygdala doesn't mess around; it's like your brain's personal alarm system. It goes off like a siren, and in a split second, it's raining stress hormones, like adrenaline and cortisol, inside your body. These little guys are like the emergency pit crew, prepping you for the "fight or flight" show. Things start to spice up from here because the amygdala is part of your limbic system, like your brain's emotional control center. But it doesn't work in isolation; it's got deep connections with the higher brain, your neocortex. The neocortex is where all the rational thinking goes down.

But the catch here is that our amygdala is under attack in our wild, fast-paced digital world. The digital realm is poking the amygdala with a stick, sometimes even hijacking its connection with the neocortex, the rational brain. It's like a sudden, "Uh-oh!" moment. And you know what happens when your amygdala goes into action mode? Your heart starts pounding like it's doing a drum solo, your palms get sweaty, and your breathing goes shallow and rapid. You're ready to sprint like Usain Bolt if you need to. So, next time you feel like your heart's about to jump out of your chest or you're sweating bullets because of a scary email, know it's your trusty amygdala at work. It's like the brain saying, "Get ready, something's up!"

As individuals, we often take our health for granted, prioritizing career and financial pursuits over our well-being. We may indulge in unhealthy eating habits, neglect regular exercise, and work late into the night, all of which can harm our health. While focusing on external success, we unintentionally donate our health to the demands of the capitalist world. It's essential to take time for ourselves, spend time with family and friends, and stay connected to society. Ignoring these things can lead to a lot of stress, which isn't good for our health. Stress can make us more likely to have health problems. Being social and living a calm and peaceful life can help us deal better with any health issues due to our genes.

We can learn something interesting from the Japanese way of living called "Ikigai." People who follow this way of living tend to live long and healthy lives. They live in tune with nature, balance things, and focus on being kind to themselves and others. Neglecting our bodies, like eating unhealthy food or not getting enough sleep, can harm us from the inside. So, eating right, sleeping well, and staying active are important to keep our body and mind healthy. Making time for ourselves, our relationships with family and friends, and our connection to society is essential. Neglecting these aspects can accumulate mental stress, activating various disease risk factors. Being a people person and leading a peaceful lifestyle can help us cope with genetic abnormalities better. In the context of healthy living and disease prevention, the Japanese practice of ikigai offers valuable insights. People following ikigai have been known to live long lives, often up to 105 or 107 years, without serious diseases. The practice emphasizes living in harmony with nature, following its laws, and maintaining a balance with our surroundings and peers. Spiritual practices, too, promote non-harm and peaceful coexistence with oneself and others.

When we neglect our body and take it for granted, engaging in unhealthy habits or excessive greed, we create a milieu that harms us from within. Proper food timing, adequate sleep, and regular exercise are crucial for maintaining a healthy body and mind. Engaging in recreational activities such as music, dance, or yoga can have a healing effect, benefiting not only our physical body but also our mental well-being. Music, in particular, has a profound impact on the Mind, and individuals fond of music often experience improved healing, especially during recovery. Surrounding ourselves with positive environments and vibrations can also contribute to the healing process.

So, if we take good care of ourselves, follow a balanced and natural way of living, and do things that make us feel good, we can keep ourselves healthy and have a happy and satisfying life. Our health is essential; making the right choices ensures we stay well and enjoy life to the fullest. In conclusion, by prioritizing our health, adopting natural and harmonious living practices, and engaging in activities that promote well-being, we can protect our most valuable asset and lead fulfilling, healthy lives.

Now, as we read together, we're learning many different things, and there's still plenty more we need to figure out. Here's a little something I want to share, and maybe you'll find it helpful too – it's called the "Serenity Prayer." It goes like this:

Dear God,

"Give me the wisdom to accept the things I can't change."
"The strength to change the things I can"
and
"The wisdom to know the difference."

It's like a reminder to help us navigate twists and turns.

GLOSSARY OF ABBREVIATIONS IN THE CARDIOLOGY BOOK

1. **AED:** Automated External Defibrillator - Portable device delivering an electric shock to restore normal heart rhythm.

2. **AFIB:** Atrial Fibrillation - Irregular, rapid heartbeat leading to potential complications like stroke.

3. **AFL:** Atrial Flutter - Abnormal heart rhythm characterized by a fast, regular heartbeat in the atria.

4. **ARVD:** Arrhythmogenic Right Ventricular Dysplasia - Inherited disorder causing ventricular arrhythmias and sudden cardiac death.

5. **AT:** Atrial Tachycardia - Rapid heartbeat originating in the atria.

6. **ATP:** Adenosine Triphosphate - Cellular energy currency involved in physiological processes.

7. **BMI:** Body Mass Index - Measure of body fat based on height and weight.

8. **BMR:** Basal Metabolic Rate - Calories the body needs at rest for basic functions.

9. **BRUGADA SYNDROME:** Genetic disorder causing abnormal heart rhythms and an increased risk of sudden cardiac arrest.

10. **CABG:** Coronary Artery Bypass Grafting - Surgical procedure improving blood flow to the heart.

11. **CAC:** Coronary Artery Calcium - Quantification of calcium in coronary arteries, indicating atherosclerosis.

12. **CAD:** Coronary Artery Disease - Narrowing or blockage of coronary arteries, leading to reduced blood flow to the heart. Also called IHD.

13. **CEPS-AC:** Certified Electrophysiology Specialist in Adult Cardiology - Certification for expertise in cardiac electrophysiology in adults.

14. **CHADSVAC:** Risk stratification tool for stroke in atrial fibrillation, considering multiple factors.

15. **CHB:** Complete Heart Block - Impaired electrical signal transmission between the atria and ventricles.

16. **CKD:** Chronic Kidney Disease - Gradual loss of kidney function over time.

17. **CIED:** Cardiac Implantable Electronic Device - Devices like pacemakers and defibrillators implanted for heart rhythm control.

18. **COPD:** Chronic Obstructive Pulmonary Disease - Progressive lung disease causing breathing difficulties.

19. **CPRT:** Cardiopulmonary Resuscitation - Emergency procedure restoring blood circulation and breathing.

20. **CPVT:** Catecholaminergic Polymorphic Ventricular Tachycardia - Rare genetic disorder causing life-threatening arrhythmias.

21. **CPR:** Cardiopulmonary Resuscitation - Emergency life-saving procedure to restore blood circulation and breathing.

22. **CT ANGIO:** Computed Tomography Angiography - Imaging technique visualizing blood vessels, often coronary arteries.

23. **CTCA:** Computed Tomography Coronary Angiography - Imaging assessing coronary artery condition.

24. **DOE:** Dyspnea on Exertion - Difficulty breathing during physical activity.

25. **DANCAVAS:** Danish Cardiovascular Screening Trial - Randomized controlled trial for cardiovascular screening.

26. **DLC:** Differential Lung Capacity - Measurement of lung function.

27. **DYPNEA:** Difficulty Breathing - Condition characterized by labored or difficult breathing.

28. **ECG:** Electrocardiogram - Test recording heart's electrical activity over time.

29. **ED:** Erectile Dysfunction - Inability to achieve or maintain an erection.

30. **EECP:** Enhanced External Counterpulsation - Non-invasive treatment for angina and heart failure.

31. **EPS:** Electrophysiology Study - Test studying heart's electrical activity and diagnosing arrhythmias.

32. **ESC:** European Society of Cardiology - Professional organization promoting cardiovascular health.

33. **FAINTING/SYNCOPE:** Loss of Consciousness - Temporary loss due to insufficient blood flow to the brain.

34. **HDL:** High-Density Lipoprotein - "Good" cholesterol removing other forms from the bloodstream.

35. **HFpEF:** Heart Failure with Preserved Ejection Fraction - Heart failure with normal ejection fraction.

36. **HFrEF:** Heart Failure with Reduced Ejection Fraction - Heart failure with reduced ejection fraction.

37. **HRS:** Heart Rhythm Society - Professional organization dedicated to heart rhythm disorders.

38. **hsCRP:** High-Sensitivity C-Reactive Protein - Marker of inflammation in the body.

39. **IBD:** Inflammatory Bowel Disease - Chronic inflammation of the digestive tract.

40. **IHD:** Ischemic Heart Disease - Condition caused by reduced blood supply to the heart. Also called CAD.

41. **INOCA:** Ischemia and No Obstructive Coronary Artery Disease - Angina-like symptoms without significant coronary artery blockages.

42. **LAA:** Left Atrial Appendage - Small, ear-shaped sac in the left atrium of the heart.

43. **LAD:** Left Anterior Descending (coronary artery) - Major coronary artery supplying blood to the front part of the heart.

44. **LBBB:** Left Bundle Branch Block - Delay or blockage of electrical impulses in the left bundle branch.

45. **LCX:** Left Circumflex Artery - Coronary artery branching from the left main artery, supplying blood to the lateral and posterior regions of the heart.

46. **RFA:** Radiofrequency Ablation - Procedure using heat to destroy abnormal heart tissue causing arrhythmias.

47. **LDL:** Low-Density Lipoprotein - "Bad" cholesterol contributing to plaque buildup in arteries.

48. **LIMA:** Left Internal Mammary Artery - Artery often used in coronary artery bypass grafting.

49. **LVEF:** Left Ventricular Ejection Fraction - Measure of the heart's pumping efficiency.

50. **LVAD:** Left Ventricular Assist Device - Mechanical pump implanted to support heart function.

51. **LVOTO:** Left Ventricular Outflow Tract Obstruction - Blockage in the outflow tract of the left ventricle.

52. **MD:** Doctor of Medicine - Academic degree in medicine.

53. **MI:** Myocardial Infarction - Heart attack, often due to coronary artery blockage.

54. **MINOCA:** Myocardial Infarction with Non-Obstructive Coronary Arteries - Heart attack without significant blockages in coronary arteries.

55. **MRA:** Mineralocorticoid Receptor Antagonist - Medication used to treat heart failure.

56. **NSTEMI:** Non-ST-Elevation Myocardial Infarction - Type of heart attack with less severe changes on the ECG.

57. **NOAC:** Novel Oral Anticoagulant - Newer class of anticoagulant medications.

58. **PAD:** Peripheral Artery Disease - Narrowing of peripheral arteries, often in the legs.

59. **PCI:** Percutaneous Coronary Intervention - Non-surgical procedure to treat coronary artery disease.

60. **PND:** Paroxysmal Nocturnal Dyspnea - Sudden shortness of breath at night.

61. **PPM:** Permanent Pacemaker - Implantable device to regulate heart rhythm.

62. **PVI:** Pulmonary Vein Isolation - Procedure to treat atrial fibrillation.

63. **PSVT:** Paroxysmal Supraventricular Tachycardia - Episodes of rapid heart rate originating above the heart's ventricles.

64. **RAS:** Reticular Activating System - Neural network in the brainstem regulating wakefulness and sleep.

65. **RAS SYSTEM:** Renin-Angiotensin System - Hormonal system regulating blood pressure and fluid balance.

66. **RBBB:** Right Bundle Branch Block - Delay or blockage of electrical impulses in the right bundle branch.

67. **RCA:** Right Coronary Artery - Primary coronary artery delivering blood to the right side of the heart.

68. **RWMA:** Regional Wall Motion Abnormality - Abnormal movement of a segment of the heart wall.

69. **SHAM TRIAL:** Clinical trial using a placebo - Study where participants receive a treatment with no therapeutic effect.

70. **SGLT2 INHIBITOR:** Sodium-Glucose Co-Transporter 2 Inhibitor - Medication for managing diabetes by reducing glucose reabsorption in the kidneys.

71. **SOB:** Shortness of Breath - Difficulty breathing.

72. **STEMI:** ST-Elevation Myocardial Infarction - Severe heart attack with characteristic changes on the ECG.

73. **SVT:** Supraventricular Tachycardia - Rapid heart rate originating above the heart's ventricles.

74. **TAVR:** Transcatheter Aortic Valve Replacement - Minimally invasive procedure to replace the aortic valve.

75. **TG:** Triglycerides - Fats circulating in the blood.

76. **TIA:** Transient Ischemic Attack - Temporary disruption of blood supply to the brain.

77. **TLC:** Total Lung Capacity - Maximum amount of air the lungs can hold.

78. **TMT:** Treadmill Test - Exercise stress test to assess heart function.

79. **TROPT:** Troponin T - Protein released into the blood during a heart attack.

80. **UACR:** Urine Albumin-to-Creatinine Ratio - Test for kidney function and damage.

81. **VHD:** Valvular Heart Disease - Disorders affecting the heart valves.

82. **VSA:** Vasospastic Angina - Chest pain caused by coronary artery spasms.

83. **VT:** Ventricular Tachycardia - Rapid heartbeat originating in the ventricles.

84. **VF:** Ventricular Fibrillation - Chaotic, rapid heartbeat in the ventricles.

85. **WPW SYNDROME:** Wolff-Parkinson-White Syndrome - Congenital heart condition causing abnormal electrical pathways.

ABOUT THE AUTHOR

Dr. Ashutosh Kumar is a distinguished senior interventional cardiologist and a heart rhythm specialist. He pursued his education at Kendriya Vidyalaya in Delhi, Mount Abu, and Kanpur. His upbringing in a defense background molded him with a strong work ethic and discipline, contributing significantly to his achievements in the field.

Dr. Kumar's educational journey commenced with completing his MBBS degree from Sri Krishna Medical College in Muzaffarpur in 2002. Motivated by a passion for learning, he continued his educational journey, obtaining an MD in General Medicine from the prestigious Banaras Hindu University in 2006. His exceptional dedication was evident as he clinched the first rank in the All-India DM entrance examination in 2006 on his first attempt. Dr. Kumar chose cardiology for his specialization at the Institute of Postgraduate Medical Education and Research, Kolkata, successfully concluding his DM cardiology in 2009.

Dr. Kumar has amassed considerable expertise and attained notable achievements during his professional journey. He has occupied influential roles in academia, initially serving as an Assistant Professor in the Department of Cardiology at GSL Medical College in Rajahmundry and subsequently at Narayana Medical College in Nellore, Andhra Pradesh. Seeking to broaden his expertise, Dr. Kumar sought international exposure by completing a fellowship at the National Heart Institute in Kuala Lumpur, Malaysia. He also undertook observerships at prestigious institutions such as the German Heart Centre in Munich, Aurora Health Centre in Milwaukee, and Veteran General Hospital in Taiwan.

Dr. Kumar's dedication and commitment to excellence have earned him international recognition. He is one of only a few cardiac electrophysiologists from India to hold the prestigious certification from the International Board of Heart Rhythm Examiners (IBHRE, USA) for cardiac device specialists (CCDS) and adult Electrophysiology (CEPS-AC). He has also been felicitated as a

Fellow from world esteemed organizations such as the American College of Cardiology (FACC), the European Society of Cardiology (FESC), the Heart Rhythm Society (FHRS), and the Society of Cardiology Angiography and Intervention (FSCAI).

Presently, Dr. Kumar holds the Clinical Director of Cardiac Electrophysiology position at CARE Group Hospital in Hyderabad and Bhubaneswar. He continues to fulfill his passion for teaching and training in cardiac electrophysiology as an Associate Professor of Cardiology at the Kamineni Academy of Medical Sciences and Research in Hyderabad, India.

Driven by a strong sense of social responsibility, Dr Kumar established the Heartbeat Foundation, Hyderabad, a charitable trust focused on raising awareness about heart rhythm disorders and facilitating their treatment.

Dr. Kumar's expertise encompasses various interventional cardiology and electrophysiology procedures, including cardiac angiographies, angioplasties, pacemakers, implantable cardiac device placements, and cardiac radio-frequency ablations. He has extensive experience in 3D mapping of complex cardiac arrhythmias and ablations. Additionally, he authored the book "ECG to Ablation- A Comprehensive Guide to Cardiac Electrophysiology (ISBN-10:8119170377) for cardiologists and electrophysiologists".

Dr. Ashutosh Kumar has made significant contributions to the field through his publications in both national and international journals. He also serves as an editorial board member for esteemed journals such as Clinical Reviews and Opinions, Journal of Cardiology and Therapeutic, and Journal of Scientific & Innovative Research.

Dr. Ashutosh Kumar's remarkable achievements, dedication to his patients, and commitment to research and education have established him as a highly respected and influential figure in cardiology. His contributions continue to significantly impact the lives of his patients and the advancement of medical science.#

For further information, contact Dr. Ashutosh Kumar by scanning the QR code:

www.ingramcontent.com/pod-product-compliance
Lightning Source LLC
Chambersburg PA
CBHW030005290326
41934CB00005B/225